SIMPLE
MARATHON TRAINING

THE RIGHT TRAINING FOR BUSY ADULTS
WITH HECTIC LIVES

Jay Johnson, MS

The contents of this book are meant to supplement training for runners engaged in marathon racing. It is the responsibility of the reader to engage in training or exercise that meets their current physical fitness abilities. The training provided in this book is not meant to substitute any recommendations by a doctor. Readers should always consult a medical professional before engaging in any physical activity.

Simple Running Training is an imprint of PFB Publishing, LLC

PFB Publishing, LLC
3845 Tennyson Street Suite 105, Denver, Colorado 80212-2107
(303) 681-8433, pfbpublishing@gmail.com

Printed by CreateSpace
Charleston, South Carolina

Cover design by Adam Batliner Art & Design
450 Harrison Ave, Suite 201 Boston, Massachusetts 02118
www.adambatliner.com

ISBN-13 978-0-692677-35-3

2   4   6   8   10   9   7   5   3   1   paperback

Simple Running Training

To all of the runners who get up before dawn to train, then take care of their daily obligations with grace and enthusiasm. I commend you for your discipline, passion, and grit.

FOREWORD

In the final mile of my marathon, I rounded the last corner and started desperately looking for the unmistakable landmark that would signify the end of one of the most incredible breakthrough races that I may ever experience. In that moment, when I was in so much pain, yet never having felt more prepared for the pain, the Brandenburg Gate came into view. As I passed under the historic gate and crossed the finish line of the Berlin Marathon, I felt overwhelmed with emotion. I wanted to cry, knowing I had accomplished something that just a couple of years prior I would've never dreamt was possible. I wanted to hug complete strangers and tell them of the feat I had just accomplished. Most of all, I wanted to raise my arms and scream and celebrate that I had just finished more than fifteen minutes faster than I had ever done before!

The time displayed on my watch, which I kept checking and rechecking out of disbelief, was definitely significant. However, more important than seeing the unimaginable finish time on my watch was the pride I felt – I had finally run a marathon the *right* way. It was the first marathon in which I hadn't relied on my watch to tell me what pace to run. It was the first time I didn't completely tank in the last 10k. It also marked the first time that I felt more joy than anguish and disappointment in the final miles of a marathon. I knew in that moment that I was now a completely different marathoner than I had been before. It was an amazing feeling, one that I will not forget.

As I navigated through the finish line of that race and made my way back to the hotel, I thought of how exciting it was going to be to share this accomplishment with the person that was instrumental in making the accomplishment happen: my coach, Jay Johnson. It was thrilling to share the news with Jay as he had guided me through my journey to running a marathon more intelligently. I have always passionately pursued my running goals, and before coming to Jay I had already qualified for the Boston Marathon, but also was often injured and rarely trained at 100%.

With a 3:34:56 marathon PR, I was feeling nearly tapped out in terms of getting faster and frustrated with the marathon training process. With Jay as my coach, I have not only thrived and felt better than I ever have in training, but I have also continued to PR beyond my wildest expectations. Berlin was the first big breakthrough, but I have continued to shave time off my previous personal bests in the marathon. To date, I have taken more than 35 minutes off my marathon PR prior to working with Jay, and now boast a 2:58:13 fastest marathon time!

In so many ways, Jay's coaching methods have helped to change me for the better as a runner. The simple yet significant changes to my training that Jay has helped implement have not only led to faster race times, but have also allowed me to enjoy my running more than ever.

Gone are the days when numbers would rule my training runs. Pace, distance, miles per week—these metrics used to mean everything to me in my running. I would spend each and every run constantly monitoring the pace, using my watch to make sure I was hitting the desired paces. Jay has helped me to understand the importance of running by feel and listening to my body rather than being ruled by the watch. The change has been transformative.

It is incredibly freeing to head out on an easy run and not feel the need to keep constant tabs on the splits that are showing on the watch. It is a beautiful thing.

The confidence to run by feel is, in large part, due to the stability that has accompanied the strength and mobility work that Jay has helped me to value and practice. I wholeheartedly believe this work to be the single most important thing Jay has done to help transform me as a runner.

Prior to working with Jay, it was difficult to know how and when to do the strength work, and often I discarded it from my training in favor of running more miles. Nowadays, having been able to feel and harness the power that has come with doing the strength work, I am happy to sacrifice more miles and cut a run short in order to make sure I have enough time to get in all the non-running work. It is just *that* important to me, as I know it is what has kept me running injury-free, allowing me to take more than 35 minutes off my marathon time.

Luckily, I rarely have to shorten a run to fit in the strength and mobility work. The way Jay has laid out the marathon training, I know how much time I need to fit in the running and non-running work. As a busy, working mom, this has been the key to making the training possible. I am easily able to map out how much time I need to finish the run and strength work before I get the kids off to school, and myself off to work.

Motivated and serious runners often have a tendency to overcomplicate things. Working with Jay, I have learned that training does not need to be complicated, and no doubt this is part of why Jay's training system is called the *Simple Marathon Training* system.

The running work I do is definitely hard, but when I look back and reflect on the things that made for an incredible marathon in Berlin, and each lowering of my personal record since, I realize how simple the work really is.

I am forever thankful to Jay not only for helping me to run faster, but also for restoring the joy in my training under his guidance.

Amy Feit

CONTENTS

INTRODUCTION

Let me ask you a few questions. Are you a busy adult? Is your life hectic? Do you love running? Do you hate having to take time away from running when you have a minor (or major) injury? Do you have faith that you can run a great marathon and finish stronger than you have in the past, perhaps even running a PR?

I've written this book for busy adults who lead hectic lives, and who want to train seriously, even after a less than ideal experience with the marathon. This book is for you if you believe you have it in you to run a great marathon when the gun goes off, and you're willing to put in the right work to make it happen.

While I've coached at both the collegiate level and the professional level, this book is inspired by my years of coaching adults, both online and in person, who have each had to find time to fit in training around their demanding lives. The Simple Marathon Training system (SMT) that you will learn in my book draws from years of experience helping adults train intelligently while they also meet all of their other obligations.

If you compare your life to the life of a professional athlete – training run in the morning, midday nap, a second run in the evening, a solid ten hours of sleep – your life, no doubt, looks a lot different. Yet, just as the professional runner is doing everything in her power to run to her potential, so are you.

This book will help you run to your potential, given the demands of your life. I'm going to be efficient and economical with my words in this book. This book is a quick read that gives you the information you need to follow a 20-week training cycle that will prepare you to run a great marathon. That is, to run to your personal potential with all the constraints of a busy life.

Obviously, twenty weeks is longer than the typical sixteen-week marathon training program that you can find for free on the internet. The reason for twenty weeks is simple: you need twenty weeks to properly strengthen your body for a marathon, dramatically decreasing the chance of injury.

If you're reading this and your scheduled marathon is less than twenty weeks away, you simply need to say, "I'm going to learn the SMT system now, but I won't be able to use it until my next marathon cycle, when I have a full twenty weeks to train." That said, you can learn the core strength, hip strength and hip mobility exercises by reading this book and watching the free videos at *SimpleMarathonTraining.com*. If your marathon is less than twenty weeks away, follow the training plan you have intended to follow, but know that in your next training cycle there is a system, the SMT system, that is the most effective way to get you ready to run your best marathon.

Before we go to the next section, I want to share a salient story with you. I had the pleasure of speaking at a high school coaching clinic a decade or so ago, when I was an assistant coach at the University of Colorado, Boulder. Joe Newton, the iconic boys cross-country coach from York High School (in Illinois) was speaking, and I was hanging on every word. Most clinicians spend their time talking about training at these clinics, but Mr. Newton told stories that highlighted how he works with high school athletes. At one point he said, "They don't care what you know, until they know that you care." I don't think Mr. Newton came up with this sentiment, as I've heard it countless times since, but it's powerful. I share this story with you because I knew much of the exercise physiology and training theory in this book when I was in my twenties, having run under the best collegiate distance coach in the U.S. (Mark Wetmore), and having coached for several years, as well as having earned a master's degree in Kinesiology and Applied Physiology. But I had no clue what it's like to be up all night with a sick child, only to catch the same illness myself twenty-four hours later (now, as a single father of two young girls, I do indeed know that situation).

Now I have the knowledge where I can help a client get to the next workout or long run ready to run well. I've learned to help business travelers fit in their training while not overwhelming their body. I've learned how to effectively coach a busy professional, who has gotten little sleep for several days in a row, as she finishes a big project or proposal. Coaching professional runners is in some ways easier than coaching busy adults like yourself. The only variables in the professional runner's life are training related. Training is what they're paid to do. You, on the other hand, are not paid to run. You are busy making a living *and* you want to race well. People rely on you for countless things *and* you want to race well. You don't have a lot of time to train *and* you want to race well. I get it. You have to meet your obligations, which you no doubt do, and intend to keep doing, with energy and grace; yet, you dream of stepping to the line of a marathon confident that you're going to have a great race, perhaps your best performance ever.

The SMT system will get you fit and keep you healthy, all while allowing you to be the person you are capable of being, for the people you love, and for the people that rely on you.

The one catch is that you have to trust the SMT system. If you're an experienced runner you will have to unlearn some of your training habits. Learn the system, trust the system, work the system. Do that and you will race well when the gun goes off. Ready to go? Great! Now let's go over the structure of the book.

In chapter one I will explain several aspects about both the marathon and the best way to train for the marathon that we need to agree on before moving forward. In chapter two I will share the eight ingredients (plus one) that make up the SMT system. In chapter three I will explain how these elements fit into the weekly schedule.

In chapter four I'll explain how 20-week SMT system is organized into five 4-week blocks. Chapter five is a brief intermission to check in and make sure you've understood me, before diving into the day-by-day training specifics of the 20-week training cycle.

Chapters six through ten explain the day-by-day training assignments, with specific detail as to what to do each day, how each day fits within the context of the week, and how all of this training is designed to get you to race day more prepared than ever before.

In chapter eleven I'll explain how to *execute* a great race. Chapter twelve will cover *recovery* from a marathon, one of the most misunderstood and undervalued aspects of training for the serious runner. Chapter thirteen is titled *The Self-Coached Runner* – armed with this book, you are a self-coached runner. This chapter is intended to help you navigate through the 20-week training cycle, with tips on how to make the right choices in your training, how to deal with the inevitable interruptions that will occur during training, and how to make sure that you're working the SMT system to your benefit.

There are many ways to tweak the SMT system and in chapter fourteen I will share these training modifications. Chapter fifteen is a collection of Q&As that I think you will find informative. Chapter sixteen is the Geek Out section of the book, which I will discuss in a moment. Chapter seventeen, Training Plans and Pace Tables, is devoted to alternative 20-week training cycles and for runners who want to run a half marathon during the 20-week training cycle. I will go into more detail about this in the ensuing chapters, but for now, you need to know that all of the long runs are assigned as miles, yet most every other day is assigned as a number of minutes.

A commonly asked question is: how much running do I need to be doing before I start training in the SMT system? The SMT system assumes that you are running 45 minutes or more, at least four days a week, before you begin. You need to have done at least two long runs of 8-9 miles in the past two to three weeks before you can start the SMT system 20-week training cycle.

There is an 8-week progression in the back of the book that will take you from running four days a week to the five days a week of running you'll do in the SMT system. You need to be able to run three miles and you need to be able to run up to 35 minutes once a week before you start this 8-week progression.

Another common question is, "Can I use this training plan if I've never run a marathon?" The answer is a definite yes, with a few caveats. First, you have to be doing the previously discussed volume of 45 minutes of running three days a week, and running a weekly long run of 8-9 miles. Second, ideally you have run a half marathon at least once before you start this training program (or have run 13 miles or longer at some point in your life). You can definitely use the SMT system to train for your first marathon, yet there is much to be said for having finished a half marathon before you start marathon training.

A key difference between this book and most training books is that in this book I've moved the technical aspects to the end. The Geek Out section of the book functions somewhat like end notes. Throughout the chapters of the book there will be spots where you can geek out on a certain topic. You can and will run well in the SMT system if you read none of the Geek Out topics. However, if you have the time to geek out, you can go to the end of the book and read the short Geek Out topics, then come back to the main part of the book and keep reading. The intent in writing the book in this fashion is to efficiently deliver the elemental information you need to train intelligently and run a great race, without being interrupted by a slew of technical material. That said, the Geek Out sections are not superfluous, and I am confident you will enjoy and benefit from these sections if you have the time to delve a little deeper.

While there is a glossary at the end of the book, I've done my best to explain the terms as they arrive in the text.

The final point, and perhaps the most important point if you're going to run well in the SMT system, is that you need to read the entire book, up to the Geek Out section, before you dive into the training. You will not and cannot have success in this SMT system if you do not first understand why you're doing what you're doing. No doubt there will be a runner who fails to read the book and dives right into the training. Failure to take the time to understand the rationale behind the workouts will most likely result in workouts that are not maximized. Learn before you leap. You can't follow the 20-week training cycle in this book unless you first read the book. As you will read in the coming chapters, the SMT system truly is simple, but you have to learn the system before you can work the system. The good news is that once you learn the system, you will get to the starting line confident that you are about to run a great race.

Now, it's time to begin the first chapter of the book, where we will agree on a handful of fundamental concepts that provide the undergirding structure of the SMT system.

⸺ LET'S AGREE ⸺

"Life is really simple, but we insist on
making it complicated."

— Confucius

H ere's the first thing you need to understand about the marathon. Your aerobic metabolism is responsible for over 99% of the energy needed to run a marathon. This is important for you to understand, especially if you've done track workouts where you run 10 x 400m as hard as you can, with 60 seconds of walking between the 400s. This workout challenges your anaerobic metabolism in addition to challenging your aerobic metabolism. If you did a workout like this in the middle of a 20-week marathon training cycle, you would be wasting a workout day to train an energy system (the anaerobic metabolism) that will contribute virtually nothing to your marathon performance.

The second thing you need to understand is the role of glycogen in marathon training. Glycogen is the preferred energy source for working muscles during exercise. Your body has plenty of glycogen to fuel your 5k, 10k, and half marathon races. Your body *does not* have enough stored glycogen to fuel your working muscles for the marathon. Depending on whom you ask, the body has enough stored glycogen in skeletal muscles and the liver to fuel you for roughly 18 miles. This obviously poses a critical problem for you as you prepare to run a strong marathon. How are you going to get from the 18 mile mark to the 26.2 mile finish line? One answer is that you can supplement throughout the marathon with sugars, in the form of sports drinks or gels, and you'll utilize this strategy on race day. The other answer is that while you don't have enough stored glycogen to fuel your body to finish a marathon, most runners have enough fat stores to fuel twenty marathons. If this is the case, then how do you take advantage of your fat stores to help fuel your marathon? Simple. You train your body to utilize fat as a fuel source. With the right training, it is possible for you to go from being a runner who can't very well utilize fat as a fuel source, to a runner who can run strong in the last 6.2 miles of the marathon because your body isn't completely dependent on glycogen.

I firmly believe that fat metabolism, also known as lipid metabolism, is the key for working adults to go from running marathons where they struggle to finish, or finish in a time that is slower than their 5k/10k/half marathon might indicate, to running a marathon where they finish strong and run to their potential. *This is the goal, to run to your fitness level and potential on race day.*

The question you should now be asking yourself is, "So how am I going to train my body to utilize fat as a fuel source?" The answer is twofold. First, you are going to have to run 18 miles or longer several times in the SMT system 20-week training cycle. Specifically, you will get in four 18-mile runs, two 20-mile runs, and one 22-mile run. Immediately following these runs you will be doing a series of core strength, hip strength, and hip mobility exercises. This non-running work is called SAM for Strength and Mobility work.

GEEK OUT
Read more about Your Long Run on page 170

SAM work is important because when you do it immediately following a run, you extend the amount of time your body is utilizing fat to fuel your activity.

By extending the duration of the workout, your heart rate will continue to be elevated, and your body will utilize your fat stores to fuel the SAM work. When you transition immediately from the long run into the challenging SAM work, you keep your heart rate elevated, which can, in a very general way, be compared to running another mile or two farther than the assigned run. I will discuss the concepts of doing SAM immediately following a run in greater detail later in the book, but essentially, in the SMT system an 18-mile run followed immediately by SAM work forces your body to utilize fat as a fuel source.

The second training method we will employ to help your body learn to utilize fat is that you will run at your goal marathon pace during the 20-week training cycle. Running some workouts at your goal marathon pace teaches your body to become efficient at using both stored glycogen and fat.

Now that you know that the marathon is 99% aerobic and that you need to be able to utilize fat stores to run to your potential, the next insight into marathon training is that the aerobic metabolism can be improved week-to-week, month-to-month, year-to-year. If we understand that the aerobic metabolism needs to be improved during training, then the question you should be asking is, "What workouts do I need to do to develop the aerobic metabolism?" In the SMT system you're going to improve your aerobic metabolism with a weekly workout on Tuesday and a weekly long run on Saturday. In the next chapter I will provide detailed explanation about how these two workouts improve the aerobic metabolism. The important thing is to understand that improving the aerobic metabolism is key if you want to achieve your marathon potential.

The fourth key concept is best explained by the following analogy. Imagine a car separated into just two things: the engine and the chassis. Now, imagine that your heart, lungs, and blood is your "aerobic engine." Now, imagine that the rest of your body—your skeletal muscles, your tendons and ligaments, your bones and your fascia—are your chassis. What happens to many runners is that they quickly build their aerobic engine, yet their "chassis" is not ready to handle the engine, inevitably resulting in injury at some point in their training. As my good friend and fellow coach Mike Smith, Director of Track and Field at Army, shared with me a decade ago, "Metabolic changes occur faster than structural changes." If this is true (and it is), then you obviously want to do everything you can to improve your chassis, as you improve your engine. This is where the SAM work comes into play. You will do SAM work six days a week, with the option of doing it the seventh day. If you do all of the SAM work assigned, the likelihood that you will be injured is dramatically reduced. While no coach or training program can guarantee that you won't get injured during training, the runners I've worked with not only tend to stay healthy during SMT, but their performance on race day is better because they are muscularly strong and symmetric, able to handle the intense pounding a 26.2-mile race presents, along with the twenty weeks of challenging training leading up to the race.

The last concept I need you to agree with is vitally important, especially if you've run several marathons and/or have followed several training programs: *If you want to do things you've never done before, then you have to do things you've never done before.* You have to do SAM six days a week. You have to trust that a 22-mile long run is in your best interest if you want to run well on race day. You have to be willing to do a brisk walk on Sunday to recover from the long run. You have to learn to run by feel, the first ingredient in the SMT system, introduced in the next chapter. If you want to stay injury-free, run to your potential, finish a marathon running strong at the end of the race, then you're going to have to do things that are part of the SMT system *that you've never done before.*

THE INGREDIENTS - EIGHT PLUS ONE

—————   —————

"Everything should be made as simple as possible. But not simpler."

— Albert Einstein

CHAPTER 2

RUNNING BY FEEL

1

The first concept that you must embrace in the SMT system is running by feel. What does running by feel mean? Let's first explore what it is not. Checking your watch throughout a run to make sure you're running a certain pace is not running by feel. You're relying on the watch to give you feedback. What happens with this approach is that if you're running the pace you want to be running, then you feel good about the run or workout, but if the pace is slower than you want to be running, you likely become frustrated.

A second example of not running by feel is a workout with a prescribed time. You may have a workout where you are assigned 4 miles at threshold pace, a pace you have determined from an online calculator, based on a recent race performance. You head out on your 4-mile threshold run at the prescribed pace, and again, you're either pleased with the pace you're running, or frustrated that you're struggling to run the prescribed pace, or extremely frustrated that you're running slower than the prescribed pace.

The final example of not running by feel is relying too heavily on a heart rate monitor. In this example, you're paying attention to a heart rate value throughout the run, often checking the watch every few minutes.

In the SMT system you will often be running workouts where you don't look at your watch during the run to see what pace you're running. In the first four weeks of the SMT system, none of the workouts have a prescribed pace, or a prescribed heart rate zone. Instead, you will be asked to run *steady* or run at a *challenging* pace. These terms are purposely vague, as I want you to learn the skill of running by feel. Every runner can learn to do this, and if you want to run to your potential, you need to empower yourself with this skill. Why is this so important? Because once you learn to run by feel you will no longer run too hard on your easy days. When life gets stressful, for whatever reason, and you have a run the next day, you can go out and run a workout based on how you feel that day. This allows you to leave the workout with a sense of accomplishment, rather than feeling frustrated by not being able to run the assigned paces. Learning to run by feel will help you on race day because you'll know how your body should feel in the first 10, 15, and 20 miles of the marathon. Yes, you can check your watch in the first few miles of the marathon to make sure you're not running too fast, but the majority of the race you will simply fall into the rhythm of your goal marathon pace.

While there will be workouts in the SMT system where you will have a prescribed pace, it's not until week fifteen that this type of workout appears in the 20-week training cycle, over three and a half months into the training. By this point in your training, you should be an expert in running by feel, a skill that will help you execute the first marathon pace workout.

Learning to run by feel will be a challenge, so I'll end with a few more pointers on what to do to learn this essential skill. You may be familiar with RPE (Rate of Perceived Exertion), a tool that has been used by both researchers and athletes for decades. The idea is that when running (or doing any aerobic activity) you can rate how hard you're working on a scale from one to ten, with ten being an all-out effort. For serious runners, ten would be a race effort. We won't be using RPE in the SMT system, but if you're familiar with RPE the jump to learning to run by feel will be easy.

Another way to think about learning to run by feel is to employ the thinking that my college coach, Mark Wetmore, taught us. He told us that if we were running easily we should be able to speak in paragraphs. If we ran a little faster, we would only be able to speak in sentences, and if we reached a pace where we were only capable of speaking in short phrases, we would know we were doing some serious aerobic running.

How much one is capable of speaking while running is a great way to think about aerobic training; however, most runners reading this book likely do the bulk of their training alone, so trying this "speak pace theory" out on the local city bike path is not the most convenient method to appraise pace. Which brings me back to running by feel. You simply need to take the plunge, abstain from looking at your watch, and do your best to run a pace that feels comfortable, one that you could sustain for much longer than the assignment for that day. If you have an assignment of a 60 minute easy run in the SMT system, you should be running a pace that you could sustain for 70 or 75 minutes. Bottom line is, if you want to do things you've never done before, such as running your best marathon, then you have to do things you've never done before, which in the SMT system means running by feel.

2 THE LONG RUN

The weekly long run is the most important day of the week in the SMT system. The long run improves your aerobic fitness by increasing the number and size of your mitochondria. The aerobic metabolism is responsible for producing over 99% of the energy required to run the marathon, so this is the primary reason to do a weekly long run. The long run increases the activity of the mitochondria, which means that they are more efficient at producing energy. Long runs also increase blood volume, as well as increasing the number of capillaries in skeletal muscle, and increasing myoglobin levels. The result of these three adaptations is that your body now has a greater ability to get oxygen to working muscles during your marathon.

The secondary reason, one that is quite simple, is if you want to race a long, difficult race, then intuitively, it makes sense that you gradually build up to long runs that pose a mental challenge similar to the marathon. While the first few long runs in the SMT system aren't long enough to present this challenge, the 18-, 20-, and 22-mile runs that you'll do over the course of twenty weeks will be. The final aspect of the long run (runs of 18 miles or more) is that they train the body to utilize fat as a fuel source. Let me explain.

When you exercise, your skeletal muscles depend on glycogen, stored in the muscle and the liver, to fuel the activity. You have enough stored glycogen to run approximately 18 miles. What this means is that sound training for 5k, 10k, and half marathon racing does not need to address the issue of running out of glycogen to complete the race. But the marathon is different. You simply do not have enough stored glycogen to finish the marathon. So how do you finish the race? Obviously you can take in sugars in the form of gels and sports drinks, but the best way to run a strong marathon is to teach your body

GEEK OUT
Read more about The Science of Optimizing Fueling During the Marathon on page 197

to utilize fat as a fuel source. You will be doing four 18-mile long runs, two 20-mile long runs, and one 22-mile long run in the SMT system, all with the goal of teaching your body to utilize fat as a fuel source. When you couple these long runs with the fact that you will be doing roughly 20 minutes of challenging SAM work at the end of these long runs, you have an over all stimulus that teaches your body to utilize fat during the course of the marathon.

The Long Run

I highly recommend that you read Dr. Carwyn Sharp's Geek Out on page 170 at some point. It's a great overview of the specific adaptations your body makes when you run long. While all of the Geek Outs at the end of the book are fantastic, you'll be well served to take a couple of minutes to read more about the long run.

3 CHALLENGING AEROBIC WORKOUTS

Most weeks you will do a challenging aerobic workout on Tuesday. There are a variety of workouts you'll do in the SMT system, but all of them have one common goal: to improve your aerobic metabolism. All of the workouts in the 20-week cycle are fueled almost entirely by the aerobic metabolism, which is exactly what we want in terms of a stimulus that will make you a better marathoner.

You may have done track workouts or hill workouts in past training. If so, you likely had a burning sensation in your lungs or a metallic taste in your mouth. These are indicators that in addition to fully using the aerobic metabolism to do the workout, you were also tapping into the anaerobic system and producing lactate (also known as lactic acid). Remember, the marathon is 99% aerobic. Compare this to the mile, where the race is split between the aerobic and anaerobic metabolism, with the aerobic metabolism only contributing 70-77% of the energy needed to run the race. While both the miler and the marathoner need to train the aerobic system, the miler needs to do some workouts that stimulate the anaerobic metabolism. In the SMT system we're not going to waste a day of training stimulating the anaerobic energy system because the anaerobic system isn't going to help you in your marathon, and the time it takes to recover from anaerobic workouts is, for the busy adult, often longer than the time needed to recover from an aerobic workout.

SAM - STRENGTH AND MOBILITY

4

The informed runner knows that to stay injury-free and race to her potential, some non-running work is essential. Every fitness and running magazine you see on the newsstand touts the latest core strength exercise that you should add to your workouts. I agree, a strong core is vital if you want to run to your potential, but popular exercises like the bicycle crunch can lead to a back injury. What exercises should you be doing and when should you be doing them? The answer is that you need to be doing A) core strength, B) hip strength, C) hip mobility, six days a week. We will use the acronym SAM (Strength and Mobility) to categorize this work.

If you go back to the analogy of needing a strong chassis that matches the size of your aerobic engine, it makes perfect sense that strength and mobility are needed to stay injury-free. The SAM work has another benefit. When you do the strengthening work that is part of each SAM assignment, you are subtly stimulating your body to produce more testosterone and human growth hormone. These anabolic hormones help "build up" the body. Conversely, running is a catabolic activity, an activity that tears down the body. If the training you must do to become a better runner is, to a certain degree, tearing you down, you offset the tearing down by doing SAM work, work which improves your hormonal profile.

GEEK OUT
Read more about Concurrent Strength and Endurance Training on page 174

The SAM work will follow each running workout and cross training day in the SMT system. SAM work is broken into SAM Hard and SAM Easy days. The SAM Hard will follow the workouts and long runs and the SAM Easy will follow the easy runs, Wednesday *tired legs run*, and cross training days. There is a progression of SAM work. You will start with Phase 1 and move on to Phase 2 once you've mastered Phase 1 routines.

If you're someone who has worked with a personal trainer or done a lot of running-specific strength work in the gym, you may progress quickly through the phases. Most of the clients I've worked with in the past haven't done much work that is similar to SAM, so it takes two to three weeks before they are ready to move from Phase 1 to Phase 2. If you do advance through the phases quickly, you will still stop at Phase 5. This will correspond to roughly week eleven or twelve of the training, weeks where you are doing 18-mile or 20-mile long runs.

While we always want the SAM Hard work to be challenging, we don't want to over-train following a workout or long run. After six to eight weeks of SAM work, you're going to begin to feel muscularly strong, just in time to withstand the increased weekly long run that will require a strong musculature to maintain good form throughout the run.

A key point of the SMT system is you have to value the SAM work as much as you value running. This work is a *need to do,* not *a nice to do.* I'll reiterate, if you do the SAM work you dramatically decrease the chance of injury. If you stay injury-free for twenty weeks of SMT system training, you have a fantastic chance of running a great marathon, perhaps even running a PR.

While there is no coach and no training plan that can guarantee that you will stay injury-free, there is strong evidence that doing the SAM work greatly decreases your chance of injury. SAM is part of the training recipe, not something additional that you can do when you feel like it. You can't expect to run a great marathon in the SMT system if you fail to do the SAM work. This work is binary: you either did it, or you failed to do it. Said another way, you can take the advice Yoda gives Luke Skywalker in Star Wars: "Do, or do not, there is no try."

SAM work will take about 10 minutes on your easy days, but will not take more than 20 or so minutes on the hard days, even in Phases 4 and 5. Again, value this work as much as you value your running.

Final Point About SAM

Go right into SAM following your run to keep your heart rate up and lengthen the aerobic stimulus. It's tempting, and probably part of your normal routine, to finish your run and then take 5 minutes to check your phone or chat with friends. However, with each minute you rest, you're losing some of the benefits of this work. Doing SAM right after the run is a key part of the SMT because it extends the aerobic stimulus, and, as I've previously explained, developing the aerobic stimulus is key to running a solid marathon.

LUNGE MATRIX AND LEG SWINGS

5

Most runners begin their run by simply running. The problem with this approach is that the body is not ready to handle the demands of running with a running-only warm-up. There is a very good chance that you consider your first couple miles of a run as *warm-up*. Perhaps you even do strides when you do track workouts, or strides before a race. Running to get ready for running is not ideal. What is ideal is to get your hips ready for the demands of running, and to get your body moving in all three planes of motion before you begin running. In the SMT system you will take 5 minutes before your run to do two things: 1) the Lunge Matrix 2) the Leg Swings.

Before I explain the importance of Lunge Matrix and Leg Swings (LMLS), please know that videos of all the exercises you'll need can be viewed at *SimpleMarathonTraining.com*. The five leg swing exercises are important because they not only improve hip mobility before the run, but the exercises also "juice the joint," getting the hips ready for the specific task that running requires. My good friend, Dr. Richard Hansen, a chiropractor who works with elite runners in Boulder, Colorado, says, "The process of pumping the joint is called 'imbibition.' It's the mechanical pumping of synovial fluid in and out of a joint space, and is one of the only ways for the joint to maintain normal integrity as we get older." Unless you're in your early twenties, then Leg Swings are an important part of getting ready.

The Lunge Matrix is rooted in physical therapist Gary Gray's work. The version you see in the videos is simple: five lunges that get you moving in all three planes of motion. Ideally, I want you to be an athlete first and a runner second. That is, an athlete who runs. If you've played any sport prior to becoming a runner, I want you to maintain as much of that athleticism as possible. When you're involved in most any other sport, you're moving in all three planes of motion. Not so with running. When you propel yourself forward, you're moving primarily in the sagittal plane with a bit of movement at the shoulder and hips.

As you run and your right knee comes up, your right hip comes slightly forward and twists toward the midline of your body; the left arm comes up and should twist slightly toward the midline of your body. This plane of motion is called the transverse plane, and running has a bit of transverse plane motion. While the third plane of motion, the frontal plane, is not part of running mechanics, runners who deliberately exercise the frontal plane will benefit from having a strong core, stronger legs, and a slightly reduced risk of injury. For this reason we will do a lunge in the frontal plane as part of the Lunge Matrix.

Your legs are going to be sore from the Lunge Matrix warm-up the first week or so that you do it. For this reason, we will start with just three reps of each lunge on each side, for a total of thirty lunges. You will build up to the full Lunge Matrix routine of five reps of each lunge on each side, for a total of fifty lunges. By the end of the second week (or the start of the third week) of the 20-week training cycle, the Lunge Matrix will not be a challenge, but routine.

In fact, I predict that in quick order the LMLS will be something that you view as a *need to do* rather than a *nice to do*. As I said above, the Lunge Matrix and Leg Swings only take five minutes (3 minutes and 30 seconds for the Lunge Matrix and 1 minute and 30 seconds for the Leg Swings).

Please note: If the SAM work takes between 10-20 minutes, and the LMLS takes 5 minutes, we need to be honest about the fact that you must create enough time in your schedule for not only the running work, but for the work to get ready for the run and the work after the run. This will make you a better runner and reduce the risk of injury. The SMT system works in large part because the non-running training is emphasized and prioritized alongside the running work. Please adopt the mentality that all of the training, running and non-running, is vital to racing well when the gun goes off.

EASY DAYS HAVE TO BE EASY AND INCLUDE STRIDES

6

For several years I've been blogging and tweeting this simple phrase: "Keep your easy days easy, so your hard days can be hard." The SMT system works because it does just this, allowing you to get in a great workout on Tuesdays and a great long run on Saturdays. You will only be ready to run well on these two days if the days that precede them are easy.

The key thing to remember when you're running on easy days is that you are going to recover from the workouts and long runs you're doing during the week *if* you run easy and slowly. I'm serious when I say that you cannot run too slowly on an easy day. The flip side is, you may fall into the same category of many runners I've worked with who have timed their easy days and have been frustrated when it was a struggle to run their typical pace for the easy day, or they have failed to run their easy day loop in the usual time. This sort of day is gone in the SMT system.

Let's say you had a great long run on Saturday. The assignment in the SMT system for Sunday will be a brisk walk. The problem is, you wake up Sunday with a sore throat. You go for the brisk walk in the morning and you come home feeling pretty good. However, by Sunday night your throat is really sore and you're not feeling 100%. You wake up Monday and your throat is still sore, but no worse than Sunday night. You're feeling about 85% so you decide to go for a run.

Monday is your easy day and you head out the door, you dutifully do the Lunge Matrix and Leg Swings (LMLS), and then start running. Here's the insight: you should be running 15, 30, even 60 seconds per mile slower than your normal easy day pace. Why? You're operating at 85% strength; if you keep the day easy, there is a good chance that you will wake up tomorrow for your Tuesday workout and be closer to 100% strength, ready to tackle the workout.

GEEK OUT
Read more about Should You Run When You Are Sick on page 176

In this example, there is the deception of feeling great while you're running, feeling great in the hours after the run, but feeling worse later in the day. Don't do this to yourself. Run easy and be back to full strength sooner.

Now that you're willing to run easy on your easy days, the second thing you need to do is to run strides every easy day. What is a stride? A stride is a short bit of running at a given pace, almost always faster than race pace. When I use the term stride, I mean something different for milers than I do for marathon runners. For marathoners, strides are going to be done at a relatively slow pace, approximately 5k race pace. You will start doing 5 x 20-second strides with 60-90 seconds easy jogging as the recovery. We will work up to 5 x 30-second strides with 60-90 seconds recovery by week nine. You will do the strides as part of the day's time assignment, which means that if you have 45 minutes assigned, the strides are part of the 45 minutes (and not done at the end of the 45 minute easy run). The very first day of the 20-week training cycle is as follows:

> M   LMLS, 45 minutes easy with 5 x 20 second strides at 5k pace (60-90 seconds easy recovery), SAM Easy.

The strides and recoveries will take between approximately 6-8 minutes. I recommend doing the strides around the 30-minute mark of the run, on a safe surface (not icy or on asphalt with gravel on top) so that you still have 5-10 minutes after the strides to run easy. Don't make the mistake of running 45 minutes, then doing your strides at the end of the run, which is how strides are done in many training programs. Better to be efficient with your easy day and do the strides in the middle of the run, allowing you the time to complete your SAM work following the run.

Why strides? The first reason is that a marathon runner should be able to run a decent 5k race in the middle of marathon training as the 5k is 97% aerobic. The rhythm of a 5k is not much faster than a marathon, yet you will have slightly different biomechanics when running 5k pace: knee lift will be a bit higher, arm swings a bit more exaggerated. You will be running a 5k in the fourth week of the 20-week training cycle, and while you will not have done any 5k-specific workouts leading up to this race, the race will help you get comfortable with the rhythm of 5k running.

Another important reason you need to do strides on your easy days is that you will feel better on your Tuesday workout and your Saturday long run having done strides the day before. You do not have any workouts at 5k race pace in the 20-week training cycle, so the fact that your legs "turned over" a bit faster the day before, means that the pace in the workout or long run will feel easier than if you had not done strides the day before.

To Summarize

1. Easy days have to be easy, so when in doubt, slow down.

2. Strides, just like LMLS and SAM, are not negotiable. You have to do your strides on all of your easy days so that the workout or long run the following day feels better. I should also note that some runners assume that doing strides on an easy day will stress their body in such a way that the day is closer to a hard day than an easy day. This is absolutely untrue. Trust the SMT system. Do your strides on your easy days and you will soon see that strides fit perfectly on the easy day, and you will often finish your easy day feeling better after having done the strides.

RUN FIVE DAYS A WEEK BUT BE ACTIVE EVERY DAY PER WEEK

7

You only need to run five days a week to run a solid marathon performance. To take it a step further, I've coached numerous athletes who have run PRs in the marathon running just five days a week, many of whom had been running six days a week prior to being coached with my training methods. That said, you need to be active every day of the week. One day a week you will do some easy cross training (biking, swimming, and elliptical are the best choices). Difficult work like P90X, TRX, hot yoga and the like do not fit the definition of easy cross training. *Easy* is the key word. On Sundays you will go for a brisk walk. You won't see a brisk walk in other marathon training programs, but my clients, after just a few weeks of doing the brisk walk, always comment about how good they feel on Monday following the brisk walk. So, there you go: five days of running, one day of cross training, and one day of brisk walking.

It's fair for you to ask, "But how am I going to be ready to run 26.2 miles if I'm only running five days a week?" My response is twofold. First, in the second half of the 20-week training cycle, you're going to be doing long runs of 18, 20, and 22 miles, so you get a spike in running volume the second half of the 20-week training cycle.

The second issue is simple, and one that you might not like, but that I must be honest about. You're a busy adult, with a hectic life, which means you have a limited amount of time to train. The SMT system will help you run a great marathon while still allowing you to meet all of the obligations in your life. Do some people run more? Sure. There is a fantastic book called *Advanced Marathoning* by Pete Pfitzinger and Scott Douglas for higher mileage marathon training. The book discusses training strategy for running 70-85 miles a week and training over 85 miles a week. That's more running

> "Most of us runners don't like the word walk. Many of us come from some kind of Spartan training backgrounds. Brisk walk sessions have become leisure and pleasure for me, but in terms of athletic performance, I have found they make me stronger. My injury issues are a thing of the past. I have been an enthusiast of mountain biking for cross training, but the benefits of the brisk walk go far beyond."
>
> — Carlos José Soto

than you'll do in the SMT system, and yet some working adults can handle this volume training (with an average of 10-12 miles a day, seven days a week).

The SMT system assumes that you don't have enough time in your life to meet all of your obligations and run this amount of volume. Unless you are going to run a marathon well under three hours, you're not going to run much more than 50-55 miles a week in any given week in the SMT system, and when you do, it will be a rare week.

To summarize, the SMT system gives you the best opportunity to run a marathon that you're proud of, while allowing you to be the adult you need to be for the people that depend on you.

MARATHON PACE RUNNING

8

Marathon Pace (MP) running is an elemental ingredient in the SMT system. The most basic reason is obvious: if you want to run a given pace in the marathon, then you should practice running this pace in your training. This training principle – running the paces in training that you want to run in the race – is called 'specificity' and all good training methods, be it for the 800m, 1500m, 5k, 10k, and half marathon, have specificity as part of the training.

Here's an example of specificity in training. If you want to run 3:30 in the marathon, then you have to run 8-minute pace for 26.2 miles. This doesn't mean you head out for a run every week at 8-minute pace and see how long you can hold on. You first build your aerobic 'engine' with challenging aerobic workouts, while at the same time building your 'chassis' with SAM work after every run. There comes a time where you do need to challenge yourself with both running at 8-minute pace and doing it for a significant distance. In the SMT system you will do a great deal of MP running in the last six weeks of the training.

Running MP benefits the serious marathon runner in several ways. First, you are biomechanically learning how to run your goal marathon pace. The knee lift and arm angles associated with this pace need to become second nature. Metabolically you need to teach your body to efficiently burn both glycogen and fat while running at MP. Finally, you will be well served on race day if you can groove MP without looking at your watch, which I consider being able to run within five seconds (plus or minus) of your goal MP. You should use your watch and the mile markers on the course in the first 5 miles to make sure you are on pace; however, you'll have a better experience if you can groove MP from that point on and not need to look at your watch.

You will not see MP assigned in the first fourteen weeks of the 20-week training cycle, but you will see it in virtually every workout and long run from the Week Fifteen point on. The reason is that you first need to get aerobically fit and structurally strong before you can profitably focus on MP.

Training at MP for several weeks will likely be a new experience for you. I often have clients who wonder if we are doing too much MP running in the final weeks of the 20-week training cycle (in part because they are getting a bit bored with the pace). Trust the SMT system and trust that you need a great deal of MP running to be able to hold the pace for the distance of a marathon.

AIF ROPE STRETCHING

+1

If you really want to be serious about your training then you need to do some flexibility work, also known as stretching. The question is, what type of stretching? Should you do static stretching or dynamic stretching? Which stretches should you do? The big question you probably have is: how much time will I need to devote to stretching? These are all great questions. Let's start with the type of stretching that you should be doing.

Active Isolated Flexibility, a flexibility method made popular in the running world by Phil and Jim Wharton, is far and away the best use of your time if you want to have the flexibility necessary to train at a high level. Most of the stretches involve a rope, so I will refer to this work as "rope stretching" though you don't need a rope for all of the stretches.

There are several routines, some taking as little as 10 minutes, others taking 20 minutes. The full stretch, which works the entire body, is 40 minutes. If you're serious about staying healthy, and you're serious about running to your full potential on race day, I highly recommend adding rope stretching to your training. You can purchase videos at *WhartonHealth.com*. You can buy a rope from *WhartonHealth.com* or purchase a rope from your local hardware store. Ninety percent of runners need an 8 ½ foot rope. A runner well over 6 feet tall needs a 10 foot rope. But, as Phil says, you can use a dog leash, or a towel, or a long sleeve t-shirt to do most of the stretches.

Rope stretching is a lot like the LMLS warm-up. The first couple of weeks will be challenging, perhaps even awkward. But, for most people who commit to doing the work every day that they run, the benefits are fantastic, and they feel much better the following day on their run. Professional athletes such as Boston Marathon champion and Olympic medalist Meb Keflezighi rope stretch several times a day. My favorite aspect of rope stretching is the breathing component.

After numerous attempts over the course of twenty years, I've never been able to do yoga, even when I work with extremely capable teachers. That said, I love the breathing aspect of yoga and the mindfulness that goes along with it.

When you are doing rope stretching correctly, you are breathing out when you lengthen the muscle, and breathing in as you release the lengthened muscle. After a few minutes, you're *in the zone*, moving your body in rhythm with your breathing, which is a great way to end a workout, or start the process of calming the nervous system before you go to bed.

GEEK OUT
Read more about Active Isolated Flexibility (AIF) on page 178

There you have it: the eight ingredients plus one, that make up the SMT system. In the next chapter I explain the rhythm of the week, what days you do workouts, what days you do long runs, what days are easy days, etc. I've alluded to the rhythm of the week up to this point, but now it's time to see not only how the training week is organized, but how one week of training sets up the following week(s) of training.

RHYTHM OF THE WEEK

—— —— ——

"Competitive sophistication (rather, complication masked as sophistication) is harmful, as compared to the practitioner's craving for optimal simplicity."

— Nassim Nicholas Taleb

I n the most basic terms, this is the structure of most every week of the 20-week training cycle:

M	Easy run and strides
T	Challenging aerobic workout
W	Tired legs run
Th	Cross training
F	Easy run with strides
S	Long run
Su	Brisk walk

When you get back to Monday you're ready for another good week of training because you're recovered from the long run.

Monday is easy, just an easy run and strides. Tuesday is a challenging workout, with SAM Hard immediately following the workout. Wednesday is often a slightly longer run, but if you make the right choice, then it is not a hard day because the assignment is to run easy, just getting in the time on your feet. Thursday is an easy, relaxed cross training day, a day that is crucial in the SMT system because you're recovering from three days of running. Friday is another easy day, just like Monday. Combine Thursday and Friday and you will be rested and ready for a fantastic long run on Saturday. The long run is the focus of each week and you need to be ready run it with vigor. Because you've had two easy, relaxed days prior to the long run, you are fully prepared to run a great long run. Because the long run on Saturday is a challenge, Sunday needs to be a day of rest and recovery. A brisk walk on Sunday allows you to recover from Saturday. This brings us back to the easy run and strides on Monday. A brisk walk on Sunday followed by an easy day on Monday allows you to be ready to run a solid workout on Tuesday. And the rhythm repeats.

Now, let's go deeper into each day of the schedule to see how the training fits together.

The SMT system is organized in an easy-to-remember seven days. There are other ways to organize training, by ten, fourteen, or twenty-one day cycles, for example. Professional athletes often organize their training in something other than a seven-day schedule. But life tends to be organized in a seven-day rhythm, so let's coordinate your training with your life. Sound good?

Roughly 90% of athletes who use the SMT system will start their week with an easy day on Monday. In chapter fourteen I will discuss how to tweak the SMT system to have you start on a day other than Monday. Monday is the best day to start the seven-day system because when you fast forward to the weekend, it allows you to run your long run on Saturday, which is, for most adults, slightly better than running the long run on Sunday.

M	Easy run with Strides

Monday starts with LMLS, which stands for Lunge Matrix (LM) and Leg Swings (LS). You simply need to watch the video at *SimpleMarathonTraining.com* to learn this warm-up routine that takes a brief, but important, five minutes to complete.

After completing the LMLS you head out for an easy aerobic run. An *easy run* means as slow as you need to go to feel good, a concept that I discussed in the previous chapter. Specifically, if you have fatigue in your legs from the long run you ran the previous Saturday, this is an indicator that you need to go slower than normal. You're running for minutes here, not miles. If you have a certain loop that you run on your easy days, then be prepared to run it one, two, or even three minutes slower than normal on a day you don't feel up to snuff. The total running workout will be between 45 minutes and 55 minutes. You will not go over 55 minutes on your Monday run, yet you will need 70-75 minutes for this workout, as the LMLS takes 5 minutes and the SAM work on your easy days takes 10 minutes. The SAM on Monday will always be SAM Easy.

Here is how the workout will appear in the training plan for Monday week one:

> M   LMLS, 45 minutes easy with 5 x 20 second strides at 5k pace (60-90 seconds easy recovery), SAM Easy.

By Week Seven you will be doing the following: LMLS, 55 minutes easy with 5 x 30 second strides at 5k pace (60-90 seconds easy recovery), SAM Easy. Between Weeks One and Seven you will gradually increase the time spent running and the duration of the strides. Remember, the five strides come as part of your run, so you will want to start them at roughly the 30 minute mark of the run to ensure that you have enough time to finish the run with 5 minutes of easy running. The strides will take roughly 6-8 minutes, depending on how much recovery you take between them.

> T   Challenging Aerobic Workout

Tuesday starts with LMLS and ends with SAM Hard. There are a variety of workouts you'll do in the SMT system on Tuesday. In chapters six through ten, I will explain each Tuesday workout. The important point here is that you need to be ready to run a challenging workout and follow the workout immediately with challenging SAM Hard work. I firmly believe that you need to *keep your easy days easy, so your hard days can be hard*. This is one reason you will finish your Tuesday workout with SAM Hard.

The challenge that new athletes face on Tuesday is simply having the mental focus to do challenging SAM work after a challenging running workout. You will do SAM Hard after hard workouts and it will be challenging physically and mentally. The good news is that after a few weeks of doing SAM Hard after your Tuesday workout, you will build the mental capacity to do this work each week, and this will pay dividends for you at mile 20 of your marathon. Obviously there will be a Tuesday, perhaps once every four weeks,

GEEK OUT
Read more about The Importance of Strength and Mobility on page 180

where you have to focus to get the SAM Hard work done, yet most weeks you will simply view SAM Hard as part of the running workout portion of the day.

The total time you spend exercising on Tuesday, from the LMLS, to the running workout, to the SAM Hard, takes longer to complete than Monday. Tuesday's running assignment, usually assigned in minutes, is longer, so this is part of the reason, but SAM Hard also takes longer.

Plan on 10-15 minutes or so to complete Phase 1 and Phase 2 of SAM for the SAM Hard routines; in Phases 3, 4, and 5 of SAM, the SAM Hard routines will take you roughly 20 minutes. This means that you need to plan your life in such a way that you have enough time to do Tuesday's workout and SAM Hard work. You don't want to feel rushed, since Tuesday is the second most important day of the week. If this means you need to get up earlier, then please get up earlier. If you need to leave work 20 minutes early, leave work 20 minutes early. If you can't leave work early, then you need to move back the rest of your evening 20 minutes to allow for the extra work. You will have a better workout if you're not stressed about getting in the workout.

If you are rushed on Tuesday, you will likely do the run and forego the SAM work. Recall that SAM is a *need to do,* not *a nice to do.* If you want to stay injury-free and race to your potential, then you need to do SAM each day that you run. Again, SAM Hard will be both a mental and physical challenge after you've done your Tuesday workout, but countless runners have done it before you, and you can do it too. Mental focus is the key here. If you're focused mentally, you can complete the physical part.

W	Tired Legs Run

Wednesday is my least favorite day in the SMT system for the simple reason that it is the easiest day for you to make a mistake in your training. The reason to do a slightly longer *tired legs run* on Wednesday than you do on easy Monday is twofold. First, you're getting in a nice aerobic stimulus with a run that is longer than your easy day. Second, when your body adapts to this run, and you feel strong and energetic on Wednesday runs, you know that you have adapted to the overall training demands of the week. Running well on Tuesday, running strong on Wednesday, then having a great long run on Saturday, most often equates to a great marathon come race day.

The difficulty with the Wednesday *tired legs run* is that if you feel fatigued on the run then you need to make sure you run easy, very easy. The worst thing you can do on Wednesday is show up to the run fatigued, then run a pace that is faster than your easy day pace and become even more fatigued. As you will learn in a few paragraphs, the focus of each week should be the Saturday long run. While you might assume that having Thursday and Friday to recover from Tuesday and Wednesday would be enough time to run a solid long run on Saturday, this is not necessarily the case. Many of my clients have run poorly on the long run on Saturday after having run a Wednesday *tired legs run* too fast. *Don't make the same mistake – when in doubt, run easy on Wednesday.*

If you look closely at the progression of both the volume and the intensity of the Wednesday run, you will see that it is very conservative. More importantly, after the first two weeks of training, there is always the option to run just 60 minutes. Please, please, be honest with yourself about how you feel, and make the right choice if you feel just average, or if you feel fatigued. In these two situations, you simply get in 60 minutes on your feet and feel good about yourself (and reap the physical benefits too). You will maintain fitness and give yourself the best chance to run well on Saturday's long run.

Depending on which week of the SMT system you are in, you are allowed to run longer than 60 minutes on Wednesday. In Week Four the assignment is: LMLS, 60-65 minutes easy, SAM Easy. If you feel good, run 65 minutes. The same holds for Week Twelve, where the assignment is: LMLS, 60-90 minutes easy, SAM Easy. In this scenario you can run up to 90 minutes if you feel great, yet you shouldn't run more than 60 minutes if you feel a little flat.

I think of Wednesday as the day that, in terms of difficulty, is between an easy day (Monday and Friday) and a challenging day (Tuesday and Saturday). It's less important than Saturday's long run and less important than Tuesday's workout, but the Wednesday *tired legs run* is part of the SMT system for a reason. We're simply trying to get in another workout that gives a subtle challenge to the aerobic system.

As with the first two days of the week, on Wednesday you'll do LMLS to start. Then you will run the assignment, always in minutes. You will end with SAM Easy. You've done SAM Hard the day before, so SAM Easy today should, just as the name implies, feel easy. As always, you need to start SAM Easy immediately following the run.

Th	Cross training Day

This is a day in the SMT system where you do some sort of cross training. This is the second easiest day of the week. After an easy run and strides on Monday, a challenging Tuesday workout, and a Wednesday *tired legs run*, this is a good break from the pounding of running. The assignment will be anywhere from 45-60 minutes. You do need to do SAM Easy after cross training, and because you may very well be doing your cross training in a public gym, be prepared for some funny looks when you're doing the hip strengthening and hip mobility exercises.

Today's goal is not to gain aerobic fitness, but rather to maintain the fitness you're gaining on Tuesday, Saturday, and Wednesday. More importantly, you're getting blood flow to muscle cells that have been damaged in the previous three days.

The key to Thursday's cross training day is that it is easy compared to all of the running days. For instance, you are welcome to bike on Thursday, but it's got to be such an easy bike ride that when you begin your run the next day, you feel refreshed. Clients who are tri-athletes, or cyclists, have a hard time riding gently on Thursday. If you have experience on a bike you need to make sure you keep this day very easy.

Biking is not the only option. Elliptical is another option, but again, you need to keep it under control. Lap swimming is one of the best things you can do on this day. Aqua jogging is great as well, though you could do 10-15 minutes less than the assigned 45-60 minutes. 30 to 35 minutes of aqua jogging is enough for Thursday. Stair climbing is too much quad dominant work for Thursday, so stay away from it.

Yoga can be a good option or a bad option, depending on the class. The test here is: does it feel easy? If you feel refreshed and recovered when you start your run on Friday, then the yoga you did on Thursday was fine. But, if you're in a "hot yoga" class on Thursday and you feel fatigued on Friday, then you've made a fixable mistake. You've gone too hard and you need to find a different yoga class! You want yoga to be restorative. It's worth noting that a yoga class will usually produce lower heart rates than other activities mentioned. This fact does not disqualify yoga as an activity for your cross training day, but rather something to be aware of when choosing your cross training activity. Forty-five minutes of biking may do a better job of maintaining your aerobic fitness compared to a 55 minute yoga class.

A brisk walk or a gentle hike is another option for Thursday. The brisk walk is mandatory on Sunday and I will explain the method of the brisk walk method soon – a unique ingredient in the SMT system.

Please don't consider running on Thursday. Cross training on Thursday is part of the SMT system for a reason, and if you decide you should run on Thursday, then you're not adhering to the system. When you work the system, you'll get to the end of the 20-week training cycle ready to run a great marathon. So, cross train on Thursday, and keep the cross training easy. Trust that you will maintain the aerobic gains you've made running.

F	Easy Run with Strides

Most Fridays will replicate Monday. You will do LMLS, followed by a run with strides, finishing with SAM Easy. The minor change you will see in the SMT system when you compare Monday to Friday is that Friday may be 5-10 minutes shorter than Monday, depending on how difficult the Saturday long run will be. This is to ensure that you are ready for the long run the next day.

Most Fridays you will feel good, having had the cross training day on Thursday, though it's not uncommon to feel flat on a Friday run. No worries, just run the assigned number of minutes, get in the strides, and remember that there is a very good chance you will feel raring to go the next day. Which leads us to Saturday's long run, the most important workout of the week.

S	The Long Run

In many training programs the long run is an afterthought. You'll see a long run in the training, but it's less important than the other workouts in the training schedule. Not prioritizing the long run is a huge mistake for the serious marathoner. The long run is the most important aerobic stimulus in terms of improving your aerobic engine. It's also the best way to prepare for the mental challenges that the marathon distance presents. If you need a refresher on the physiological importance of the long run, simply go back to chapter two.

The long run is assigned in miles, which is obviously different than the days leading up to this run. You will build your long run distance through the 20-week training cycle, starting at just 10 miles in Week One and gradually progressing to a run of 22 miles in Week Sixteen. There is only one 22-mile long run in the 20-week training cycle, and it's critical that you get this run in.

The progression of the mileage from week-to-week in the SMT system is sound and will allow you to safely run longer and longer each week, until you reach the serious long runs of 18, 20, and 22 miles. On many of the long runs you will have the option to speed up in the last few miles of a run. Only do this if you feel strong. Do not try to force a long run, but rather, let the run come to you.

You may have heard the terms *progression long run* or a *fast finish long run*. Neither of these terms apply to our long run schedule. The SMT system long run is either A) an easy run where you are just getting in the distance, or B) a run where, if you feel well, you can speed up a bit in the final miles of the run. Speeding up means that you subtly increase your pace, then maintain that pace for the last few miles of the run. There is nothing set in stone in terms of a pace assignment, as the assumption is you will soon learn to run by feel in the SMT system and be able to gauge if you should speed up or not. Specifically, by Week Five, you should be able to run by feel, which means that the 13-mile long run should go well, with you finishing the run saying you could have run at least one more mile at the finishing pace.

Key Point

In every long run in the SMT system, you need to be able to say, "I could have run one or two more miles at my finishing pace if I had to." This is true for the shortest run, the 10-mile run, you do in Week One, and it's also true for the 22-mile run you do in Week Sixteen. You should be able to say, "I could have run 23 miles today, but I'm so glad I didn't have to."

The key to the long run is that you make the right choice in terms of running by feel and running a pace that you can maintain for the entire run. Here are some examples of making the right choice when it comes to the long run.

First, you need to get the time in on your feet. If you are getting in the volume assigned, then you are getting in a quality aerobic stimulus, regardless of the pace. This means you can run an easy pace on the days you feel flat. Goal number one with every long run is simply to complete the mileage that is assigned.

Second, if the schedule says that you should speed up at the (fill in the blank) mark of the run "if you feel good," then please do so. But, the key here is to be honest with yourself about how you feel. If you are a bit fatigued, then don't change pace. Getting in the time on your feet is more important than running a bit faster in the last few miles of the run.

Finally, you should be running with good posture throughout the run. The long run is a great time to practice running with good posture. Because you will be fatigued at the end of the long run, you are particularly susceptible to employing poor posture. You want to run with a slight forward lean, a lean from the ankles to the shoulder, not from the hips to the shoulders. Many runners start to lean forward at the hips when they fatigue. Biomechanically this causes a braking force as the lower leg (called the shank by biomechanists) has a positive angle. We want the lower leg to be as close to perpendicular with the ground as possible when running.

Following the long run, you need to get a drink of water or a few sips of a recovery drink right away. However, this must be done quickly, in less than sixty seconds, because you need to go right into SAM Hard. As I shared with you earlier in the book, doing SAM Hard immediately after the long run has several benefits and the only way to take advantage of the elevated heart rate aspect of SAM Hard is to start it as close to the end of the long run as possible.

What often happens for runners in the SMT system is that the long run is going well and they're running strong, and in the last mile they think, "I'm having a great run, but soon I'll be done and I have to do the SAM Hard routines. I don't know if I have the energy to do that." Please, reverse this self-talk and say, "I'm having a great run and when I finish I'm going to knock out the SAM Hard work with the same energy and focus that I've had in this run." It is worth recalling that one primary reason to do SAM Hard work immediately after a hard run is for the mental challenge that mimics the mental challenges of a marathon. You do four 18-mile runs, two 20-mile runs and one 22-mile run in the 20-week training cycle. That's eight opportunities to run a significant long run and then have the mental discipline to focus for roughly 20 more minutes. What a great way to prepare to run to your potential on race day. Remember, SAM Hard following your long run will be extremely challenging, but you can do it!

The final point I need to make about doing SAM Hard work after the long run is simply that I have been asking athletes to do challenging, non-running work, much like SAM hard, for over a decade, and the results are unequivocal. After several weeks of adapting to the mental challenge of doing rigorous non-running work following the long run, athletes gain fitness rapidly. There is research showing that strength work following endurance work can increase mitochondrial density. As my fellow coach, exercise physiologist, and friend Dr. Jeff Messer says, "As distance runners we're

GEEK OUT
Read more about You Do Hard Things on page 182

in the business of building mitochondria." Learning about this research was extremely exciting to me, because for years I have seen that athletes who did work very similar to SAM Hard after their workouts made great improvements in their racing. I thought it was just a function of the improved running economy (RE) that comes with strength work, a connection that has been shown several times by different research labs.

To think that strength work improves the aerobic system was surprising, and yet empirically I had seen the correlation, without knowing the causation. Now we know that not only does the challenging musculoskeletal work following a run improve a runner's hormonal profile, it also improves the aerobic engine by producing more mitochondria.

Most runners want to do the weekly long run on Saturday morning as it allows them to enjoy the rest of their weekend. Think about this for a moment. In Week One you will be doing a 10-mile run, yet in Week Twelve you will be doing a 20-mile run. Over the course of three months you have to carve out twice as much time to get in the run (plus your SAM Hard will take a few minutes longer following the 20-mile run). The long run will take a large chunk out of your Saturday, and in the second half of the 20-week training cycle, you're likely to want a nap at some point following the run. The most successful clients I work with have supportive families and/or supportive significant others, who understand the importance of the long run and are happy to help them get in an afternoon nap.

Meeting a group for a long run is well worth the organization it will require. That said, the one problem with group runs is that you must run the correct effort and not run with someone who is running a bit faster than you need to run. A difference of 10 seconds a mile is a 2 minute difference over 12 miles and 3 minutes over 18 miles. This is not insignificant, so be very careful if you're meeting a group for a long run. The other issue is that when you do your SAM Hard immediately after the run, you will get some strange looks, and potentially receive some ribbing from your fellow runners. Don't worry, most of them will have some sort of setback or injury in the coming months (sorry, it's true), and after their setback or injury, will likely ask you what you do to stay injury-free. Your comeback will be, "It's probably the funny-looking exercises I do at the end of my runs."

Su   A Brisk Walk

Sunday's brisk walk assignment is one of the key differences between SMT system and other training programs. It's crucial for your recovery and a great way to spend time with a non-runner significant other who has missed you while you have been out running. Kids in strollers and dogs will love joining you for the brisk walk too! It's a win-win, if there ever was one.

Many clients initially resist the idea of a brisk walk because the assignment is at least 45 minutes and could be as much as 75 minutes or 90 minutes. Clients who do this work see the obvious benefits after just a few weeks. Your legs feel better by the end of the brisk walk and you have a better run on Monday when you do the walk. You ran the hardest workout of the week just twenty-four hours earlier. On the cellular level, you have damaged muscle fibers from the long run, and the best way to help repair this damage is to get oxygen-rich blood to those fibers. Think of the brisk walk as a necessary recovery activity, allowing you to be fully ready to run a great workout 48 hours later, on Tuesday.

Pushing children in a stroller or taking an active dog for a walk are the two ideas I had in my mind when I initially added this element to my clients' weekly training. Some clients go for a gentle bike ride, or a hike, and those are fine, yet, as with Thursday, you need to make sure that you keep the overall workload low on Sunday.

Other clients use this time to make a phone call to friends or family, while others catch up on their favorite podcast. I even have a client who, during the brisk walk in a local state park, takes a photo or two of the native flora. If that feeds your soul, great, so long as you get in the brisk walk.

Brisk does not mean going out for a stroll. You should definitely be able to cover 3 miles in an hour when you walk briskly, assuming you're walking in a flat area. Flat is the best walking course to take, but gentle rolling hills are good too. Many clients cover close to 4 miles in an hour on a brisk walk.

Take note: don't plan to feel good in the first 10, 15, or 20 minutes of the walk, but you should feel good by the end of the walk. If you don't, you may want to shorten Monday's run by 10-15 minutes.

Clients often wonder why they're not going for an easy run on Sunday. The answer is simple. You don't need to run six days a week to run a great marathon. If you try to run six days a week the chance of injury increases. The SMT system will get you to the starting line fit and ready to run a great marathon, with you running just five days a week. The brisk walk is the same as all of the other ingredients in the SMT system, it's a *need to do*, not *a nice to do*.

SAM Easy is not mandatory on Sunday, but you will increase your chance of staying injury-free if you do SAM Easy on Sunday.

Summary Of 7-Day Training Week

Monday is an easy run with strides, followed by SAM Easy. Tuesday is a solid aerobic workout, followed immediately by SAM Hard. Wednesday is an easy run followed by SAM Easy. Thursday is 45-60 minutes of easy cross training. Friday is the same as Monday, an easy run with strides and SAM Easy. Saturday is the most important day of the week – the long run. Sunday is a brisk walk, 45 minutes to 1 ½ hours.

OVERVIEW OF THE 20-WEEK TRAINING CYCLE

—— ——

"Simplicity is the
ultimate in sophistication."

— Leonardo da Vinci

CHAPTER 4

Before I go into detail about each week of the 20-week training cycle, I want to give you an overview of the training, broken into five 4-week periods.

WEEKS 1–4 LEARNING THE SYSTEM

The goal of the first 4-week period is simply to learn the SMT system's rhythm and to start the process of learning to run by feel. You will have four weeks to do this, culminating in a low-key 5k race. The 5k race is part of the SMT system for two reasons. First, it's simply fun to get out and race, especially since you'll train for sixteen straight weeks following the 5k. Second, it's great to get a sense of your fitness at the outset of the 20-week training cycle. While online running calculators have many flaws, we will use your 5k time to get a projected time for the marathon. The goal with this is simple. If you can stay injury-free and get in all of the assigned training between the 5k in Week Four and your marathon in Week Twenty, I am confident that you can run faster than the time projected. Why? Because you'll gain fitness on Tuesday and you'll gain fitness on Saturday, and the SAM work will keep you healthy. Combine improving your aerobic engine with the consistency of training injury-free and you have a recipe for your best marathon come race day.

The one thing you need to be honest about in the first four weeks of training is: *if you want to do things you've never done before, then you've got to do things you've never done before.* This is your new mantra. Mantras are made for repeating, and you will repeat this mantra over many a mile in the next twenty weeks, and thus perform to your potential in the marathon.

If your marathon training hasn't been great in the past, or you've had problems 20 or 22 miles into a marathon, and you want to have a better experience in both your training and on race day, then you need to trust the new elements you'll do in the SMT system. LMLS and SAM are important, and running by feel is a must if you want to race to your potential. You need to make the long run the focus of each week, which may or may not have been your focus in past training cycles. A brisk walk on Sunday is not a throw away day, but rather a day where you recover from the long run and start the process to prepare for a great workout on Tuesday. *If you want to do things you've never done before, then you have to do things you've never done before!*

WEEKS 5-8
LEARNING TO WORK THE SYSTEM

In the second 4-week block of training you'll be doing three things. First, you'll be increasing your long run volume. Because the long run is the most important day of the week in the SMT system, we need to prioritize the progression of the long run. In Weeks Five, Six, Seven, and Eight, the run is 13 miles easy, 14 miles easy, 14 miles where you can speed up at the end if you feel good (different than the previous 14-mile run), and 16 miles easy. The jump from 14 miles to 16 miles is a very safe jump. Why not 14, 15, then 16? I've found that when an athlete can run a certain long run distance and speed up the last few miles, this is a better indicator that they are ready to increase the long run distance rather than just completing the run. That said, the first goal of every long run is to simply complete the distance that is assigned. Most runners are able to speed up in the second 14-mile run, running a faster pace in the last 3 miles.

The second thing that changes in the second 4-week block is that the Tuesday workouts become more challenging. Don't worry, you'll be able to handle this change because at this point A) you are fairly good at running by feel, which you'll need to learn to run these workouts well, and B) you've done SAM Hard work four times after a Tuesday workout, so you know what to expect in terms of SAM Hard being both a mental and physical challenge. In Week Six, you'll do your first Yasso 800s workout, a workout I'll describe in detail in chapter seven. You'll do three Yasso 800 workouts during the 20-week training cycle. This will be a day when you want to go to bed earlier than normal and you'll want to give yourself plenty of time to finish the workout. I'll go into detail about how much time you will need for this workout in chapter seven.

The final element that changes in the second 4-week block of training is that the SAM Hard routines and exercises will be challenging for you. If you start at Phase 1 SAM in Week One, then by Week Five you should be on Phase 2 of the SAM work. At the other end of the spectrum, if the SAM work is only moderately challenging, there is a chance that you are starting Phase 3 of the SAM work in Week Five. Phase 3 of the SAM work is challenging for most runners, even if you had good levels of general strength before you start the SMT system. Regardless of where you start, you will be doing SAM Hard after your Tuesday workouts and Saturday long runs.

WEEKS 9–12
SERIOUS TRAINING
PART 1
WELCOME TO THE
LONG RUN

In the third 4-week block of training, the SMT system starts to really challenge you. I'll get into the details in a moment, but first I want to say that there is a big difference between the first eight weeks of the SMT system and the remainder of the 20-week training cycle. The difference is simple: You can get away with less sleep and poor dietary choices in the first eight weeks of training, but starting in this third block of training, these lifestyle habits will start to catch up to you as the training becomes much more intense. Tuesdays are challenging and Saturdays are long, and you need to be well-rested and properly fueled if you're going to handle the training from here on out.

GEEK OUT
Read more about The Latest Sleep Science on page 183

The first big change in the third 4-week block of training is that the long run is 16 miles in Week Nine and 20 miles in Week Twelve. Between these two runs are two 18-mile runs. The first 18-mile run is just to get in the time on your feet, while the second 18-mile run you should speed up just a bit in the last 3 miles if you're feeling strong.

By now you know the importance of the long run. What you now need to understand is that the difference between a 16-mile run and an 18-mile run is not just a 2-mile increase. For example, the jump from a 14-mile run to a 16-mile run is not nearly the challenge that jump from a 16-mile run to an 18-mile run is. This is why you need to be well-rested and giving your body great fuel in the form of nutrient rich food. If the jump from 16 miles to 18 miles is challenging, the jump from 18 miles to 20 miles is even more challenging. You'll only run 20 miles twice in the SMT system 20-week training cycle. Be rested and ready for the first 20-mile run in week twelve.

The Tuesday workouts in this third block of training are formidable. That said, you are ready to handle these workouts, so long as you A) run easy on Monday, and B) make sure you get a good night's sleep on Monday before the workout. SAM Hard is challenging in this block of training for the simple fact that both the long run and the Tuesday workouts are more difficult. You'll run hard in the workout Tuesday and then you'll run a solid long run on Saturday. In both scenarios you have to go immediately into the SAM Hard work and knock it out. Be ready to bring energy and focus for an additional 20 minutes after the run.

Wednesday may very well tend toward the longer end of the 60-90 minute spectrum. However, please remember this: if you feel average or poor at the 45-minute mark of a Wednesday run, make the right choice and run 60 minutes. Wednesday is such a tricky day because if you feel strong, you can and should run a bit longer. In this block of training you're allowed to run 70, 80, 85, and 90 minutes over the course of the four weeks. Yet, a key to the SMT system is that you make the right choice on Wednesday, which means you only run more than 60 minutes if you feel strong and energetic. Be honest with yourself on Wednesday, and make the right choice.

The good news about the third 4-week block of training is that now you know the system, and you're ready to really work the system. You know what to expect in terms of what the goal of each day of training is. You're going to challenge yourself twice a week, and you're also going to get two easy days of running twice a week. Trust the system, work the system, and begin believing that you can run a great marathon come race day.

WEEKS 13-16
SERIOUS TRAINING
PART 2
MOST CHALLENGING
FOUR WEEKS OF
TRAINING

The fourth 4-week block is no doubt the toughest block of training in the SMT system. You are still five to eight weeks away from race day. This is not the time to rest, but rather, it is time to improve your fitness so you can run a great race two months down the road when the gun goes off.

Let's start with the long runs. The long runs are 18, 18, 20, and 22 miles during these four weeks. Every run is important, every run will be challenging, and following each run you will have to be both focused and energetic to do the SAM work. These are four great opportunities to teach the body to utilize fat as a fuel source. You've got to do your best to make the physiological adaptation, and this is the critical block of training where you will have the training opportunity to do this.

In the first 18-mile run, if you're feeling well, speed up just a bit for the last 4 miles. You'll get to the 13 mile mark and take inventory of how you feel. If you feel strong and energetic, speed up when you get to mile 14. If you feel average or poor, maintain pace, get in 18 miles and knock out the SAM Hard work, and feel good about the day.

The 20-mile run in Week Fourteen is an opportunity to both get in the 20 miles and to speed up a bit in the last 3 miles of the run. That said, the number one goal is to get in 20 miles on your feet; if you can't speed up the last 3 miles, simply finish the run, knock out the SAM Hard work and feel great about your long training day. You should finish this run saying, "I could definitely have run one more mile today, perhaps two."

The next 18-mile run is very challenging. The goal is to run 6 miles at marathon pace (MP) within the run. You'll run the first 11 miles easy, then MP from mile 11-17, and easy for 1 mile to the finish. It's an extremely challenging day. It's also a day that I consider to be the second most important long run of the 20-week cycle, after the 22-mile run.

The good thing about the 22-mile run is that it's simple: 22 miles at an easy pace (start a few seconds a mile slower than your normal easy pace for long runs) and finish saying, "I definitely could have run 23 miles today, but I'm glad this is over." You'll do SAM Easy following this run because we don't want to overwhelm you with both the longest run of the 20-week cycle and SAM Hard. Because this run takes such a toll on your body, the three days following the run are a brisk walk, a complete day of rest and a 45-minute run with strides. By the time you get to Wednesday's run you should feel recovered.

There you go, four long runs in the fourth block of training. While these runs are indeed quite challenging, take heart! You will be able to complete them and feel strong doing so.

Next, I have a few thoughts on goal marathon pace (MP), a crucial aspect of sound marathon training. Of course, you don't go out and run 26.2 miles in training as hard as you can. Along the way we will take data from your training that indicates your fitness and what pace you can reasonably expect to run for a marathon at the end of the 20-week schedule.

You most definitely need to do some running at the projected MP to prepare your body for the specific demands of this pace over 26.2 miles. You'll do a lot of MP running in the final weeks of the 20-week training cycle. In fact, there is so much MP pace work as you get closer to the race, that I often get comments from clients, such as, "I'm getting a little sick of MP, but I trust that I need to do it." Trust it. These same clients run great races on race day and much of this is because they have *grooved* the rhythm of MP into their training.

So how do we know what your goal marathon pace should be for the race? Simple. You'll be doing your last Yasso 800s workout in the fourth block of training. Assuming you have a decent-to-good day, you'll simply use the corresponding formula and give yourself a conservative estimate of the finish time you should be shooting for. Use the table in chapter seventeen to determine your MP based on your average splits from the Yasso 800s workout.

It's important that you get in enough MP running in both this block of training and the final block of training. This means that some of the Tuesday workouts will have you running MP over an assigned number of miles. With this in mind, you'll need to figure out how long these workouts are going to take you. If you have 8 miles at MP and you're running 7 minutes per mile, the run will only take you 56 minutes. If you're someone who is trying to run 3:55 for the marathon, just under 9 minute mile pace, the run will take you just over 70 minutes. Make sure you take the time to do the math as to how long your Tuesday workout will take you. Rarely do I have clients who fail to account for how long these Tuesday workouts, based on miles, will take, but it has happened.

The final point I want to make about the fourth 4-week training block is that SAM Hard after the Tuesday workouts and the Saturday long runs is going to be very challenging. There is no need to progress the SAM work in this 4-week block unless the SAM Hard you are doing is exceedingly easy for you.

In this block of training, the workouts and long runs are the most difficult that you've done up to this point, and doing SAM Hard immediately following the run is going to be challenging. You're ready, and remember, you do hard things so that you can do things you've never done before. Use the self-talk, "You do hard things," when you're grinding through the SAM Hard work, remembering that you're getting a psychological benefit from this work as well as a physical benefit. You're improving your capacity to stay focused when your body is uncomfortable and this is a great skill given how uncomfortable you're going to be in the final miles of the marathon.

WEEKS 17-20 GROOVE MARATHON PACE TO HAVE A GREAT RACE

This is both a challenging and delicate block of training in the 20-week training cycle. By the time you get here, you'll be ready for it! The final 4-week block of training will prepare you for race day.

The first thing we need to talk about and define is the word *taper*. I'm going to use this word, but I want to be clear that the term taper means different things to different people, just as the term stride means different things to different people. In the taper we simply want your legs to become more refreshed as you get closer to the race, so that on race day your legs can handle the specific demands of running 26.2 miles at MP. However, we don't want you to lose any of the aerobic fitness that you've worked so hard to gain over the past four months. So, what to do? We will gradually lower the volume you're running, shorter long runs for instance, but we won't lower the intensity, keeping some MP running in the long runs. This is a classic coaching concept: decrease volume, but keep intensity relatively high. I wish I could take credit for this concept, but I certainly cannot. The best coaches in the world use this formula to get athletes ready to perform at their best on race day.

Now, let's see how the taper plays out in the workouts and long runs. As with the previous 4-week cycle, you need to be prepared for longer workouts because most of the Tuesday workouts will be assigned in miles. The long runs will gradually decrease in distance in the final four weeks of training. You'll run 16 miles, 14 miles, 12 miles, and finally you'll run the race. All three of the long runs have MP running as part of the run, yet the amount of MP running decreases as the length of the run decreases.

Key Point

The huge mistake that many runners make in this final 4-week cycle is running 6 or 8 or 10 miles at MP and saying to themselves, "How in the world am I going to be able to run this for 26.2 miles?" You must erase this negative thinking from your mind. If you trust the SMT system, you're going to be able to run your goal MP on race day. You must trust that the combination of your fitness, your ability to utilize fat as a fuel source, and your fresh legs will culminate in a great marathon. It takes faith, no doubt about it. Silence the negative thoughts and simply get in the MP work that is assigned. If you do this, you're good to go.

Because you're a busy adult with a hectic life, there is no doubt that you could use more sleep. Do your best to try to get just 10-15 more minutes of sleep each night in this 4-week block of training. This amount of sleep, while it may seem trivial for just one night's sleep, will compound into you being more rested, more energetic, and more positive about your ability to run 26.2 miles. You also need to eat as many nutrient-rich meals as you can. You might have heard the term "eating clean" and this is exactly what you want to do. This said, don't be sparse with your diet. You're still training at a high level and you have to bring in enough fuel to support your training. If you want more information on how to get to a healthy race weight by race day you can read Matt Fitzgerald's book *Race Weight*.

Remember, we want your legs feeling fresh; said another way, we want your legs feeling *poppy*. The one potential problem with this is that when you go out and do strides, both on your easy runs and also in your pre-race (the day before the race), you can easily slip into running the strides faster than normal. Be mindful of this tendency and make sure your strides in this last 4-week block of training are no faster than they've been in the preceding weeks. Your legs should feel good and you should want to run faster, but hold yourself back and just cruise through the strides.

Related to this is that when we talk about *race day* in chapter eleven, I'll discuss the importance of running MP in the opening miles of the race.

Because your legs are rested and feeling fresh, there is a strong tendency for most marathon runners to get caught up in the excitement and energy of those around them and run 5, 10, or 15 seconds a mile faster than their MP in the opening miles of the marathon. Please, don't do this. You compromise all of the work you've put into your race if you make this mistake. Simply run your MP. When you do this, you get to mile 20 ready to grind out the last 6.2. Your mantra on race day is *groove and grind*. Groove MP for 20 miles and grind the last 6.2.

GEEK OUT
Read more about Using Imagery To Run Your Best Marathon on page 187

One of the most important aspects of race week is imagery. Imagery is simple, doesn't take a lot of time, and can have a huge impact on your race. You can do it anywhere, anytime. Yes, you can do some of it on your runs, but ideally you create a bit of time in your day for imagery.

There you go, a 20-week training cycle broken into five 4-week blocks of training. Each block progresses into the next, with the simple end goal being you running a great marathon when the gun goes off on race day. Trust the SMT system, work the system, rest well, and eat well so that you are ready to run to your potential on race day.

—— INTERMISSION ——

"Clarity is power."

— Buckminster Fuller

CHAPTER 5

Wow! We've covered a lot of ground in the introduction and the first four chapters. You've had the opportunity to identify if this is the right system for you (if you are a busy adult and your life is hectic, then it is). You know that the marathon is 99% aerobic and that you don't have enough stored glycogen in your skeletal muscles and liver to finish 26.2 miles, which means that you need to teach your body to utilize fat as an energy source. You also know that you need to *strengthen your chassis to handle your aerobic engine*, and you will be doing SAM work at least six days a week to do so. You now understand *if you want to do things you've never done before, then you have to do things you've never done before.* The SMT system has elements that are no doubt new to you, and the SMT system is either missing or de-emphasizing elements of training that you have done in the past. You need to trust the system, and you need to work the system if you're going to run a great race come race day.

If you want to become a better runner you need to learn to run by feel. If you want to become a better marathoner then you need to emphasize the long run as the most important day of the week. You need one challenging aerobic workout each week to improve your aerobic fitness. The SAM work is a *nneed to do,* not *a nice to do.* Six days a week you'll do SAM and you need to trust that this work will not only decrease the chance of injury, but will help you handle greater volumes of training and greater intensities of training in the second half of the 20-week training cycle.

The Lunge Matrix and Leg Swings (LMLS) take a total of 5 minutes and you must do these exercises before every run. Your easy days need to be easy (which you will be able to execute since you will be learning to run by feel) and need to include strides. You'll run just five days a week in the SMT system, but you will be active seven days a week. Trust this balance of hard days and easy days as the most intelligent way to maximize the time you spend training. Remember, if you were a professional runner, or if your life were less demanding, you could train differently. The SMT system is for people like you: busy people with hectic lives. Finally, if you can make time for Active Isolated Flexibility (rope stretching) you can take another huge step towards both decreasing the chance of injury and increasing your ability to handle longer, more intense workouts, and long runs.

You now know what to expect each day of the week. Said another way, you understand the rhythm of the week, and how one week sets up the next week of training, so that week after week you're gaining fitness toward the goal of running a great marathon.

Monday is an easy run with strides followed by SAM Easy. Tuesday is a challenging aerobic workout, followed by SAM Hard. Wednesday is the *tired legs run*, followed by SAM Easy; this is the day that you need to be honest about how you feel and vigilant about making the right choice. Thursday is an easy cross training day that ends with SAM Easy. Friday is essentially the same as Monday, though you will often run 5 to 10 minutes less on Friday to be ready for the Saturday long run. Saturday is the most important day of the week because on this day you will run your long run (unless you've arranged to shift your training schedule, which is covered in chapter seventeen). Get to bed at a reasonable hour on Friday so you can maximize your effort on Saturday. The SAM Hard you will do after the Saturday long run will be both physically and mentally challenging, but you can do it, so stay positive. Sunday is a brisk walk, the day you won't see in other training programs. After a few weeks of doing a brisk walk following the Saturday long run, you'll be a convert to brisk walking because your body will feel so much better going into Monday's run.

Note

You can shift the seven days in either direction, but you have to keep the order of *easy day with strides*, followed by *challenging aerobic workout*, then *tired legs run*, in the same order of progression as I've just laid out. I will go into detail about how to tweak the SMT system in chapter fourteen.

You now know what the 20-week training cycle looks like. You know that the twenty weeks are organized into five 4-week blocks of training.

In the first 4-week block you're simply learning the SMT system, specifically learning to run by feel. You'll end this block of training with a 5k race. In the second 4-week training block you're doing three things: building the length of your long run; accomplishing Tuesday workouts that are more challenging than the first 4-week block of training; completing challenging SAM Hard work on both Tuesday and Friday.

In the third 4-week block of training you enter what I would term *serious training*. You're doing long runs of 16, 18, and 20 miles. These runs require both good aerobic fitness and a great deal of mental focus. SAM Hard should be done immediately following these runs, which means that your total physical and mental output for the day is very high. Tuesday's workouts are challenging as well, and again, you must do the SAM Hard work immediately following the workout. Wednesdays get longer and become a significant aspect of the week's training. The good news about this block of training is that you know how the SMT system works, so now you are simply working the system to become a better runner. You are moving towards race day, gaining fitness each week. This is a challenging but very rewarding block of training.

As you know by now, the toughest 4-week block of training is the forth block of training. Your long runs are 18, 20, 18, and 22 miles, with the second 18-mile run comprised of 6 miles at marathon pace (MP) in the middle of the run. You have to be sleeping well and eating well to maximize these runs. You can do this. You can prioritize the Saturday long run in your life in such a way that you have plenty of time for your run and can also enjoy the weekend with friends and loved ones.

The 22-mile run is a focus, and it is the only time in the 20-week cycle that you are asked to run this distance. Don't forget that the MP running that you will do in this phase of training will be challenging as well. Make sure you have enough time on Tuesday to get in your MP running and not be rushed to finish the workout. Finally, SAM Hard is assigned twice a week, once following the Tuesday workout and once following the Saturday long run. SAM Hard will pose the most difficult post-run challenge you have faced so far in the 20-week cycle. You're ready to physically do this work after running hard, so long as you are mentally prepared to do the work.

The final four weeks of the 20-week cycle will prepare you to run a great race. Don't overthink the training at this point. Simply look at the training, do it, then turn off your head. You need to silence the voice that says, "I just ran 10 miles of MP and it wasn't easy – how in the world am I going to run 26.2 miles at that pace on race day?" Erase this kind of thinking and trust the SMT system. There is a huge focus on MP work in the last four weeks of training. While many of these workouts mix it up by having you run a fast pace in the middle of the workout, you need to put in the work and run your goal marathon pace.

You have to teach your body the rhythm of goal marathon pace. You need to *groove* marathon pace into your muscle memory so that on race day you have a simple plan: *groove* the pace for 20 miles, *grind* for 6.2 miles. *Groove and grind* is the name of the game come race day and all of the MP running that you do in the final 4-week training block prepares you to execute this simple race plan.

There you go, a brief summary of all that we've covered to this point. Which brings us to chapter six, the part of the book that you'll use as a reference throughout your training. In chapters six through ten I will give an overview of the assignment for each day of training with specific descriptions of each element. The descriptions will explain how you need to approach a workout or run, how each workout or run fits within the context of the week or within the 20-week training cycle, as well as what pitfalls you need to be mindful of to make sure you have a profitable workout. Use chapters six through ten as a reference to come back to as often as needed.

The SMT system is not complicated. Yes, there are many elements that go into it, but you now know what those elements are. Now, it's time to see how the elements fit together and play out day-to-day in the 20-week training cycle.

TRAINING WEEKS 1-4:

LEARNING ——— THE SYSTEM

"It is the effort to improve that is valuable. By repeating it over and over you will master it."

— Shunryu Suzuki

CHAPTER 6

Week 1

In Week One the goal is to start the process of learning the SMT system. Given that you are running 45-minute runs and long runs of 8-9 miles before you start the SMT system 20-week training cycle, the amount of running you'll do the first week will be very doable. That said, you will start the process of learning to run by feel during the Tuesday fartlek workout, and this can be challenging. Simply get in all of the work this week – LMLS before you run and SAM after you run – and don't worry about how sore you may be from this work. By Week Three, or perhaps Week Four, the soreness will be gone and your legs will feel strong.

Note: Just 3 reps of lunges on each side this week for all LMLS warm-ups.

M   LMLS, 45 minutes easy with 5 x 20 second strides (60-90 seconds easy recovery), SAM Easy.

T   LMLS, 10-minute warm-up, 30 minutes of 3 minutes on, 2 minutes steady fartlek, 10-minute cool-down, SAM Hard.

W   LMLS, 50 minutes easy, SAM Easy.

Th   LMLS, 45 minutes easy cross training, SAM Easy.

F   LMLS, 40 minutes easy with 5 x 20 second strides (60-90 seconds easy recovery), SAM Easy.

S   LMLS, 10 miles easy, then immediately into SAM Hard.

Su   Brisk walk of 45-60 minutes, LMLS before and SAM Easy afterward is encouraged.

The week starts on Monday with the Lunge Matrix and Leg Swings (LMLS), then a 45-minute easy run and 5 x 20 second strides, followed by the Strength and Mobility (SAM) Easy routine.

The best way to learn the LMLS is to watch the videos at *SimpleMarathonTraining.com*. LMLS takes just 5 minutes. You're not following the SMT system if you skip the LMLS. Doing the LMLS to start every run gives you a better chance of staying injury-free during the training. You will be sore the first few days you do the LM portion, and for this reason you will only do three reps on each leg for each of the five lunging exercises. Three reps of five lunges on each leg is a total of thirty lunges each time you do the LM in Week One. In Week Two you'll up to four reps on each leg (for a total of forty lunges). In Week Three you'll do the standard five reps on each leg (for a total of fifty lunges). In the SMT system you will not do more than five lunges on each leg for each type of lunge, so you won't do more than a total of fifty lunges before you go for a run. Don't be intimidated by the soreness you'll likely experience this first week doing the LM. Right now, you're likely weak in your lower body and core. The LM will help you gain the needed strength in both areas.

One of the two or three most important elements of the SMT system is that you must run your easy days at an easy pace. What is "easy" running? Easy is just like it sounds. It's a pace that you could run for a couple of hours, even at this early stage in your training. You can never run an easy day too slowly, but you can run an easy day too fast. This is important: you're not gaining fitness on your easy days, but rather maintaining the fitness that you currently have. While you could argue that you are gaining fitness on your easy days, for the purpose of this book we can assume that the gains you make on easy days are much less impactful than the gains you'll make on Tuesday and Saturday.

Over the course of the next twenty weeks you will no doubt have a few assigned easy days when you're tired and you don't feel strong and energetic. If you're running the easy days correctly, on the days you don't feel strong and energetic, you may be running 30-60 seconds a mile slower than your normal easy day pace. That said, you might run 15-20 seconds per mile faster on a couple of easy days in the coming weeks if you feel great. There is no need to check your pace during the run. The first Monday you will run 45 minutes and strides, which I'll explain next. On Friday you will only run 40 minutes and strides to make certain you feel good for Saturday's long run.

What does *45 minutes with 5 x 20 second strides (60-90 seconds easy recovery)* mean? Let me explain. Every time you see *5 x 20 second strides* you run the strides at 5k pace and take 60-90 seconds of easy running/jogging as recovery. You don't need to time these strides each week, but it's not a bad idea to look at the paces on your GPS this first week to make sure you're running 5k pace and not any faster. After the first week or two of doing strides you won't need to look at your watch; instead, simply run by feel. These strides are done as part of the run. If you run 45 minutes, then you probably want to start your strides at the 30-minute mark of your run. The strides will take roughly 6-8 minutes to complete, so you will have at least 5 minutes at the end of the 45-minute run to go easy.

The reason to do the strides is simple: you should always be able to run a decent 5k in the middle of marathon training. To run a good 5k you need to have some 5k pace running in your training, even if it is just 20 seconds at a time. The second reason to do strides is the neuromuscular stimulus you get from this type of work. The term neuromuscular describes the nervous system's interaction with the muscles. Many busy adult runners fail to include any neuromuscular work in their training. This is a mistake, but one that is easily corrected by doing strides on your easy days.

When you do strides at 5k pace on Monday before your Tuesday workout, the pace of the Tuesday workout feels easier. Why? Your legs remember the 5k pace from the day before, and because the pace of most Tuesday workouts is slower than 5k pace, the Tuesday workout pace is perceived as pleasantly manageable.

I often get the question, "But if I'm doing strides, then doesn't that mean that the day is harder than an easy day?" Absolutely not. As you'll learn, in the SMT system, strides won't make your easy day any harder than doing an easy run. 90% of the time you feel good doing the strides, even if you feel so-so in the running leading up to the strides.

Following the run you need to complete SAM Easy. Start with Phase 1 of the SAM work. All of the videos you need for SAM are on *SimpleMarathonTraining. com*. I won't describe each exercise and each routine, as they are described in detail in the videos. If it seems like a lot of information the first time watching the videos, don't get overwhelmed. Once you do the routines a few times you'll have them memorized. If you want to download a PDF with all of the exercises and routines, we have these on the *SimpleMarathonTraining.com* site as well.

While there is a chance that you're coming from a background where you've done a lot of work that is similar to the SAM work in SMT, please just follow the Phase 1 SAM program for the first two weeks of training. If the SAM work is too easy in the first two weeks of the training, please feel free in Week

Three to jump ahead in the SAM progression and go to Phase 3. Be patient; between the SAM work and the running, you'll be putting in quite a bit of work by Week Four of this program.

Key Point

Go right into the SAM work following your run as you keep your heart rate up and thus lengthen the aerobic stimulus. Finishing your run and taking 5 minutes to check your phone or chat with friends is counterproductive. Doing your SAM immediately after the run is a key part of the SMT because it extends the aerobic stimulus, and as you probably know, developing the aerobic stimulus is key to running a solid marathon.

In this training plan the longest run you'll ever do on the easy days (Monday and Friday) is 55 minutes. The reason to keep the run under 60 minutes is simple: we want you to be able to finish an easy day in 75 minutes, from the start of the LMLS to the end of SAM Easy. Five minutes for LMLS, 55 minutes for the run with strides, and roughly 10-15 minutes for SAM Easy, so 70-75 minutes total.

If you go straight from LMLS to the run, then right into SAM Easy, you get an aerobic stimulus that is 70-75 minutes; more than enough for you to maintain the fitness you will be gaining on Saturday's long run, Tuesday's workout, and Wednesday's *tired legs day*.

Tuesday is your first workout, a simple fartlek workout of 3 minutes *on* followed by 2 minutes *steady*. You will do this for 30 minutes, six sets total. The fartlek workout is a key workout for learning to run by feel. Why? I'll explain in a moment. First, I want you to know that fartlek workouts have been employed for decades.

GEEK OUT
Read more about Concurrent Strength and Endurance Training on page 174

The term fartlek is Swedish for speed-play. That's all you're doing with a fartlek workout. You're simply playing with different paces, alternating between faster running and slower running, making sure that the faster running isn't too fast and the slower running isn't too slow. We will alternate between two different paces in our fartleks, but a fartlek workout could involve more than two paces. For instance, you could alternate between marathon, half marathon, and 10k pace.

You may be wondering why the first workout is a fartlek workout. Fartlek workouts help empower you with the ability to assess how you're feeling when you're running faster than your easy day pace. Specifically, how much discomfort is appropriate for a given duration or distance? A fartlek can teach you this. The fartlek workouts in the SMT system are based on effort, not pace, so it is up to you to learn how to execute these workouts so that you find a balance between feeling tired at the end of the fartlek workout, yet knowing you could have done another set or two of fartlek if you had to. You can think of fartlek workouts as the precursor to more intense workouts, where the line between running hard but controlled, and running too hard, is thin.

To be clear, almost every workout in the SMT system should be run controlled. You can run hard, but you need to run controlled. I will answer the question, "How do I know if I'm running controlled?" in the chapter fifteen Q&A. Running controlled is a fundamental principle in the SMT system.

In the SMT system the fartlek workouts will have a certain number of minutes *on* and a certain number of minutes *steady*, with the *on* and the *steady* equaling 5 minutes. You will do both 3 minutes *on*, followed by 2 minutes *steady*, as well as 4 minutes *on*, followed by 1 minute *steady*, in the 20-week training cycle. If you warm-up for 10 minutes, go right into the fartlek, then cool down 10 minutes, you'll have run 30 minutes of fartlek (six sets), a nice little 50 minute workout.

4 minutes *on*, 1 minute *steady*, is definitely a challenging workout, especially for athletes who know how to execute the workout. You'll do some 4 minutes *on* and 1 minute *steady* in both Week Four and Week Seven.

Failing in your first fartlek workout is a great outcome! Why? Because running by feel is one of the most important concepts in the SMT system and *blowing up* in the workout, e.g., crumbling at the end of the workout because you ran too fast in the beginning, is a great learning opportunity. You'll do a better job executing not only the next fartlek run that is assigned, but also in next week's workout – a progression run.

Ideally, you should finish this workout saying, "I could have run one more set of 3 minutes *on*, 2 minutes *steady*, and been fine. And I could have run a second set after that, but that would have been a race effort." So, this first fartlek run is not an all-out effort, but rather a controlled effort.

Invariably, I'm asked by new clients, "What pace should I run for the *on* portion and the *steady* portion?" I don't give specific paces for two reasons. The first reason is that I don't know your fitness level and in these first few weeks of training we are simply getting you into the rhythm of the SMT system. As long as you run a challenging workout, but not a race-effort workout, you've accomplished the goal of the fartlek. The second reason I don't give paces is that I want you to learn that *steady* is not slow running. Please don't look at your watch during the workout. When the workout is over, you can look at your splits. If there is more than a 90-second-per-mile difference between the *on* pace and the *steady* pace, then your *steady* pace is too slow and your *on* pace is too fast. As you gain fitness, the difference between the two paces will begin to decrease to roughly a minute, or slightly less than a minute. For fit athletes who have a good sense of pace, the difference may come close to 30 seconds.

The first fartlek workout you'll do is 50 minutes of continuous running. Run 10 minutes easy, then go right into the fartlek. When the 30 minutes of fartlek is over, go right into the 10 minute easy cool-down, then straight into SAM Hard. SAM Hard will be challenging, so be ready for it. A 50-minute running workout is not a long workout and will only be mildly challenging mentally, but your first SAM Hard assignment will be both a physical and mental challenge. Stay focused and move through the exercises in SAM Hard. If you have to take a break between exercises, that's fine. You will have another crack at the same SAM Hard work following Saturday's long run.

Wednesday is a simple day. LMLS, then a 50 minute run, then SAM Easy. Add the three elements together and you have 65 minutes of work. In just a few weeks you will be running well over an hour on Wednesday, after having run a challenging workout on Tuesday. For this reason, this workout is called the *tired legs run*. The first Wednesday is just 50 minutes, so your legs shouldn't be too fatigued from the workout the day before.

Thursday is a cross training day. As mentioned earlier in the book, cross training days need to be easy. You need to go easy enough on Thursday that you feel fresh for Friday, even though Friday is an easy run with strides. You will do 45 minutes of cross training this week, but soon you will build up to 60 minutes of cross training. You need to do LMLS before the cross training activity, finishing with SAM Easy. You may feel self-conscious doing the LMLS and SAM work in a gym environment, with other people watching. Do the SAM work as it is your primary protection against injury.

Friday is a replica of Monday, with one minor change. You will often run 5 minutes less on Friday than Monday to ensure that you are fully ready to run well for the most important workout of the week—the Saturday long run. Make sure you get strides in on Friday, as the neuromuscular stimulus of running 5k pace makes the pace of the long run feel easier.

You need to establish good habits for your long run, and you need to do this in the first week. The first essential habit is to get up early enough before the long run to have something light to eat and something to drink. Choose foods that won't spike your insulin.

Choosing a course is important for the long run. If you're going to run a loop course you should ideally choose a loop that is 2 miles shorter than your assignment. Why? If you have a horrible run you can cut the run short by 2 miles. Again, this won't be an issue the first week when you run 10 miles, but when you're doing 18 miles (which you will do four times during the next twenty weeks) it's good to have the option of stopping at 16 miles. Long runs get exponentially harder on the body as the distance increases.

You will do SAM Hard after each long run (except the 22-mile run). It's critical that you do this work as soon as you can after finishing the run. You can get some liquids in when the run is finished, but you should go into the SAM Hard exercises following the long run for the simple reason that it extends the aerobic stimulus for the day.

I'll give you an example to illustrate the point. Let's assume we have a runner who runs 8-minute pace for the 16-mile run. Now, let's assume that the post-run SAM for the particular week will take 16 minutes. If the runner can go right into SAM Hard following the run, keeping the heart rate up, the aerobic stimulus is similar to an 18-mile run because the aerobic system was challenged for an additional 16 minutes.

The SMT system works best when you set up your space for the SAM work in such a way that you can finish the run, take a few sips of water or a low-sugar sports drink, perhaps with some protein, and go right into SAM Hard. You save your body the pounding of running 15-20 additional minutes, while getting an aerobic benefit that is similar to having run 2 extra miles. Doing this takes practice and you need to practice the first week. It also takes a high degree of mental focus to do the long run and go right into SAM Hard.

Finally, your significant others and friends need to understand that you will be running and doing SAM for a significant period of time on Saturday mornings. Runners who have a supportive family or significant other will find it easier to train at a higher level. Again, the first week you're only doing 10 miles, so you won't be gone long. This is a good week to calculate how long you'll be gone for the 16-, 18-, 20-, and 22-mile runs. Letting the people in your life know in advance that on Saturday mornings you won't be available will help your cause immensely.

You likely won't need an afternoon nap the first week, but you will certainly need a nap the day of the 22-mile run. The need for a short afternoon nap for all of the Saturday long runs varies from person to person. When in doubt, get in bed or jump on the couch and sleep for 30 minutes at some point on Saturday afternoon.

Sunday's brisk walk might seem to you like an odd assignment. You've already taken a cross training day on Thursday, so if you don't run on Sunday, you will have run five days in a week of training. Running just five days a week, but being active all seven days of the week, is a key reason why the SMT system keeps runners injury-free and increases their aerobic fitness.

GEEK OUT
Read more about The Latest Sleep Science on page 183

Why go for a walk rather than doing some other activity? First, you need to have blood moving to the lower body since the long run on Saturday causes damage to the muscle fibers that propel you forward. There are obviously other things you can do to get blood-flow to your lower body, but a walk is the most convenient way to accomplish this goal. People can leave their doors and be walking at a moment's notice. The second reason to do a walk is that the biomechanics of walking are similar to the biomechanics of running. This gives your body a chance to subtly strengthen the small muscles of the lower leg and foot, without the pounding.

You need to trust the brisk walk as a viable training day for the first few weeks of this marathon training cycle. Most of my clients question the validity of the walk in the beginning of our work together, but after a few weeks I get comments like, "I can't believe how much better my legs feel at the end of the walk."

The final aspect of the walk is that it must be brisk. Brisk walking is somewhat dependent on your height, yet even shorter athletes should be able to walk between 3 and 4 miles in an hour, assuming the course is flat. If you can walk a dog or push a baby stroller at that pace, then this is a perfect day to do so. If you have a friend or spouse that will join you for the walk, this is a bonus, but in this case, you should make sure that the walk is brisk and doesn't become a leisurely Sunday stroll. LMLS and SAM Easy are not mandatory on Sunday, but if you have the time, I highly recommend including these two elements on Sunday.

You need to follow the plan exactly as it is prescribed for the first week. If this means running with a simple watch that does not have GPS capabilities so that you're not tempted to run a faster pace on your easy days, please do. If it means that you have to endure the soreness incurred by doing the Lunge Matrix, trust that you won't be as sore in Week Two, and trust that by Week Three you won't be sore at all. If your mindset has always been to run workouts as hard as you race, please have the self-control to run Tuesday's workout at a challenging but controlled pace. You need to be able to finish Tuesday's workout saying, "I could have run one or two more 5-minute reps." If the week looks easy on paper, please just do the running and when the running ends, go into the SAM work with focus and energy. The running is easy the first week, but for most athletes, the SAM work is challenging for several weeks. Start your SAM work at the Phase 1 level. If the Phase 1 SAM is ridiculously easy, then you can bump up to the Phase 3 level, skipping Phase 2, in Week Three.

Finally, I want to share something that Bob Kennedy shared with me. Bob was the former American record holder in the 5k and the first non-African to run the 5k in under 13 minutes. He talked about "being on top of your training, not under your training."

This is a great quote to keep in mind. At no time in the 20-week training cycle do I want you to be at the absolute limit of what you can handle for training. Yes, I want you to be training very hard as we get closer to the marathon. You'll be running between 18 and 22 miles for your long runs in Week Twelve through Week Sixteen, with challenging workouts on Tuesday, plus a *tired legs run* on Wednesday. This is a lot of training, yet as Bob Kennedy says, you need to be on top of the training, always feeling like you could do a bit more. In the very first week of training you should feel like you can do much more. The experience of feeling like you can do more in training is one reason why the SMT system is so effective.

Week 2

This week you will do a progression run on Tuesday, the next step in learning to run by feel. You need to start this run at a conservative pace so that you can speed up throughout the run. Before every run this week you are going to do four reps of each lunge in the lunge matrix, which means you will do forty lunges total. Your legs may be sore, but trust that your legs will soon adapt to the work. You will run 5 minutes longer on Wednesday, cross train 5 minutes longer on Thursday, and run 1 more mile on Saturday. The increase on Saturday's long run to 11 miles may not look like much, but it's a 10% increase, and this is significant. Obviously, you wouldn't have the 11-mile run assignment if it weren't appropriate, but you shouldn't assume 11 miles is going to be easy.

Note: Just 4 reps of lunges on each side this week for all LMLS warm-ups.

M   LMLS, 45 minutes easy with 5 x 20 second strides (60-90 seconds easy recovery), SAM Easy.

T   LMLS, 10-minute warm-up, 30-minute progression run: 10 minutes steady, 10 minutes faster, 5 minutes faster, 5 minutes fastest but controlled, 10-minute cool-down, SAM Hard.

W   LMLS, 55 minutes easy, SAM Easy.

Th   LMLS, 45-50 minutes easy cross training, SAM Easy.

F   LMLS, 40 minutes easy with 5 x 20 second strides (60-90 seconds easy recovery), SAM Easy.

S   LMLS, 11 miles easy, then immediately into SAM Hard.

Su   Brisk walk of 45 to 60 minutes, LMLS before and SAM Easy afterward is encouraged.

WEEK 2

Monday's workout is the same as the previous week. Remember, run 5k pace for your strides and no faster. You will be doing four repetitions of each lunge in the LM this week. You will probably have some quad soreness this week, but it should be much less than last week. For some runners there is no quad soreness this week.

Tuesday's workout is a simple progression run. Just like last week, this is one continuous run. You run 10 minutes to warm-up, then go straight into the 30-minute progression run. You want to run the first 10 minutes of the 30-minute progression conservatively; the next 10 minutes, run a bit faster but still be very controlled; speed up more for the next 5 minutes, and even more for the final 5 minutes.

The last 5 minutes should be *fast but controlled*. It's not the end of the world if you can't speed up later in the workout, it just means that you ran too hard to start. Do not run all-out in the final 5 minutes—this is not the assignment! The assignment says, *5 minutes fastest, but controlled*. If you are running controlled at the end of the workout, it indicates that you could run at least 5 minutes more at this finishing pace, and perhaps 10 minutes more, though this would probably take you into race effort, not something we want to do at this point in the training schedule.

As with the previous week, there are no pace assignments; you need to learn how to run by feel, and it's crucial that we do this often in the early weeks of the training cycle so that you don't have any problems with pace during the longer workouts in the middle of the training cycle. Following the 30-minute progression run, go straight into 10 minutes of cool-down, then right into SAM Hard. Again, you want to keep the time between the running and the SAM Hard as brief as possible. Keeping the transition brief allows for the maximum aerobic stimulus for the day.

You may be wondering why there is no change in Week Two for the Monday and Friday easy days. At this point in time, there is no reason to run more than 45 minutes on these days to maintain fitness. Later in the training you will need to run a bit more, but even then we want to follow a simple phrase that I know is true for runners and I know will benefit you: *keep your easy days easy, so your hard days can be hard*. A simple little phrase, but it captures so much about the SMT system. Monday and Friday should never be punishing workouts. If you keep these days easy, you give yourself a better chance to have a great long run on Saturday and a great workout on Tuesday. If you run a little too fast on Monday or Friday, making the day more challenging than it should be, you run the risk of running poorly on the Saturday long run or the Tuesday workout. *Keep your easy days easy, so your hard days can be hard.*

SAM Easy should be easier by Friday of the second week. As you know, the SAM phases are designed to take roughly two weeks. So here you are, near the end of your first two weeks of training and you've done SAM Easy a minimum of five times, but SAM Hard will be a challenge following Saturday's long run. We want to challenge your musculature with each SAM Hard session in the first eight weeks of training. You need to gain muscular strength so that you can handle more running in the middle of the training cycle, as well as handle the intensity of the workouts you'll need for the marathon you are capable of.

Remember the analogy of your body being a car: your bones, muscles, tendons, and ligaments are the car chassis, and your heart and lungs are the engine. You need a chassis that is strong enough to support your aerobic engine. The catch is that you gain fitness (improve your engine) faster than you can strengthen your chassis. Put another way, the metabolic changes that come with intelligent training occur faster than structural changes. While we are building your aerobic system in the first eight weeks of training, the SAM work is just as important if you're going to stay injury-free later in the training cycle. The SMT system does a great job keeping most athletes injury-free because there is so much emphasis placed on the SAM work in the first two months of training.

Don't worry if you struggle to get through Saturday's SAM Hard exercises. You can simply repeat the Phase 1 SAM work next week (Week Three). I've had many clients do this and it is absolutely fine. As Buddhist monk Pema Chödrön says, "Start where you are." If you are muscularly weak, that's fine. We will start with Phase 1 SAM and do this until you're ready to advance. *The key point is that you're doing work to strengthen your body, in ways that you've never done before, for things that you've never done before.* Think how much faster you can run when you have a stronger physique!

Saturday you have 11 miles, just one mile longer than the week before. For most runners the distance is not a problem, but SAM Hard will be a challenge. You need to get into the habit of doing the SAM work immediately after the run. This transition isn't what you're accustomed to, so when you hit mile 10 of the run, remind yourself that you have 20-30 more minutes of work ahead of you. In the coming weeks the seamless transition between the end of the run and the start of SAM will be the norm, but today you'll need to be ready and be focused for this work.

Sunday's walk is straightforward. The key, as with all of the Sunday walks, is to keep the pace brisk. Enjoy the walk and feel good about having done two solid weeks of training.

Week 3

The Monday/Friday easy runs are each 5 minutes longer than the previous two weeks. Be ready to be mentally challenged in the Tuesday workout of 4 x 8 minutes at a challenging pace, with 3 minutes steady. You may be ready for Phase 2 of SAM Hard on Tuesday, but if you're not quite there, simply do Phase 1 and feel great about your workout. Wednesday is a 60-minute run, 5 minutes longer than last week. Saturday you will do 12 miles easy. Plan on a mental challenge of SAM Hard after this run. Sunday's brisk walk is 5 minutes longer than the previous two weeks. If you can, get in the full 65 minutes.

Note: 5 reps of lunges on each side this week for all LMLS warm-ups. This is the full LM warm-up.

M   LMLS, 50 minutes easy with 5 x 20 second strides (60-90 seconds easy recovery), SAM Easy.

T   LMLS, 10-minute warm-up, 4 x 8 minutes at a challenging pace with 3-minute steady recoveries, 10-minute cool-down, SAM Hard.

W   LMLS, 60 minutes easy, SAM Easy.

Th   LMLS, 45-50 minutes easy cross training, SAM Easy.

F   LMLS, 45 minutes easy with 5 x 20 second strides (60-90 seconds easy recovery), SAM Easy.

S   LMLS, 12 miles easy, then immediately into SAM Hard.

Su   Brisk walk of 50 to 65 minutes, LMLS before and SAM Easy afterward is encouraged.

WEEK 3

The workout on Tuesday is the first aerobic repeat workout. You'll run 10 minutes to warm-up and 10 minutes to cool down, then 4 x 8 minutes at a challenging pace with 3-minute steady recoveries. The key to this workout is twofold. First, you need to run controlled on the first two 8-minute segments so that you can speed up a bit on the third segment, and run your fastest repetition on the fourth segment. The second key to this workout is that you need to keep the recoveries at a steady pace. If you run the 3-minute recoveries at a steady pace, this workout is essentially a fartlek workout, as you oscillate between two paces. The workout is 41 minutes of solid aerobic running. As you know by now, this is a continuous run of 10 minutes to warm up, then you go right into 41 minutes for the workout, followed by a 10-minute cool-down, for a total of 61 minutes of running. You need to be able to say, "I could have run one more 8-minute segment, but it would have been close to a race effort." You do not need to finish this workout saying, "I could have run two more 8-minute segments." SAM Hard will be taxing today because you ran a challenging workout, and you will likely be doing SAM Phase 2 for the first time. Just get through the SAM Hard routines knowing that it is designed to be difficult work. As you know, you need to go right from the run into SAM Hard to get the best aerobic benefit from the day's workout.

You will run 60 minutes on Wednesday, 5 more minutes than you did the week before. You may feel fine on this run or you may feel tired and sore. Either way, the important thing is to get the time in on your feet. You can't go too slowly today. Even if you feel strong and energetic you shouldn't speed up on this run, but rather run easy and enjoy the scenery. The third week of training needs to be as low-key as possible, with the long run, the aerobic repeat workout, and the SAM work being the most challenging aspects of the week.

Thursday is a cross training day, a day that must be easy. Don't make the mistake of working too hard today, but rather use this day to recover from three days of running. If you keep Thursday easy then you'll be ready for a good run on Friday and a great long run on Saturday. You'll hear this phrase throughout the book: *when in doubt, do less* (#WIDDL).

A simple assignment for Saturday: a 12-mile long run. If you kept Thursday's cross training day easy and you keep Friday's easy run with strides easy, then this shouldn't be too difficult, even though it is a mile longer than last week. Make sure you go right into SAM following this run as this imparts the aerobic stimulus of a run that would be a mile or two longer. Keep the pace easy on this run, though there is no harm in speeding up just a bit in the last 2 miles of the run if you feel fantastic. But do not start this run with the mindset that you must speed up in the final miles of the run. Only speed up if you have run the first 9 to 10 miles feeling great.

You should always end a long run saying you could have run another mile or two at the assigned finishing pace. This is true even for your 22-mile run. Start this practice today, making sure that when you finish the run you are confident that you could have run 13 miles and felt great doing so.

Week 4

Week Four is an interesting week, as you will be running a 5k race on Saturday to determine your baseline fitness. There are 5ks every weekend in every major metropolitan area in America, so for most people finding a race won't be a problem. You may live in an area that does not have a weekend 5k race option. In this case, run a 5k time trial on your own in order to get a reasonable indication of your fitness.

M	LMLS, 50 minutes easy with 5 x 20 second strides (60-90 seconds easy recovery), SAM Easy.
T	LMLS, 10-minute warm-up, 20 minutes of 3 minutes on, 2 minutes steady, right into 20 minutes of 4 minutes on, 1-minute steady fartlek, 10-minute cool-down, SAM Hard.
W	LMLS, 60-65 minutes easy, SAM Easy.
Th	LMLS, 45 minutes easy cross training, SAM Easy. Note: Must make sure the cross training is easy today.
F	Pre-race, LMLS, 10-15 minutes easy, 4-5 x 20 second strides (60-90 seconds easy recovery) 5-minute cool-down.
S	Pre-race, LMLS, 10-15 minutes easy, 4-5 x 20 second strides, finishing the strides roughly a minute or two before the gun goes off. Execute a great 5k Race! 10-minute cool-down down jog, then SAM Easy after the race.
Su	Brisk walk of 35 to 60 minutes, LMLS before and SAM Easy afterward is encouraged.

There is an important point you need to embrace regarding this race. You will be running this 5k having done strides at 5k pace, but not having done any 5k-specific workouts leading up to the race. This is by design. Racing a 5k will give you a baseline of where your fitness is, giving a conservative approximation for your goal marathon pace, sixteen weeks from now. We will use an online calculator to get a prediction of what you can run for a marathon based on this 5k, but there are several things you need to understand that accompany this calculation. Before we talk about the calculators let's talk about your mindset going into this race.

We know the marathon is 99% aerobic; similarly, the 5k is 95% aerobic. The training you have done in the first four weeks of this marathon cycle has been solid aerobic training. You should feel good about the fact that when you race the 5k at the end of Week Four, you will have roughly a month of training in preparation to run a solid race.

There is a concept that high school, collegiate, and professional athletes often use in their training: "training through races." This means they don't take any special measures to rest for a race, other than taking the day before the race to do a pre-race routine, which makes that day shorter than most easy days. When you train through a race, you still race as well as possible, but you finish knowing that you could have run a bit faster if you had been rested. In the SMT system, we assume that you can take 10, 15, or even 20 seconds off your 5k performance due to the fact that you trained through the race, and you didn't do any 5k specific workouts to prepare for the race. But here's the key: you can't go into the race thinking, "I'm not ready to do this." You are ready to run a solid 5k, just not as prepared as you would be if racing a 5k were the focus of your training. You're in a marathon training cycle, not a 5k training cycle. We are simply using this race as a tool to help set goals for the marathon and to help figure out what pace you should run the Yasso 800s in Week Six.

After the 5k race you'll want to use an online running calculator to get a rough estimate of what you could run a marathon in at this time. Go to the *Resources* section in the back of the book for a list of calculators. When you plug a time into a calculator, the prediction is a very good indicator of what you can run for the distance directly above the race you ran. If you ran a 5k in 21 minutes and the calculator says you could run about 43:40 for 10k, then I would trust the 10k number. What you cannot trust on Saturday afternoon when you get home and plug in your 5k performance into a calculator is the estimated marathon performance. The 21 minute 5k corresponds to about 3:25 for the marathon. Can you run 3:25 sixteen weeks from now? You bet. Can you run it today? Probably not. And this is where people get into trouble. They see the number that the calculator predicts, but they don't understand the training that is necessary to get them to the goal. To run a good marathon, you need to do long runs of 18 miles or longer; you need to do marathon-pace running (and feel comfortable running the pace); you need to do a challenging aerobic workout each week; you need to do enough volume each week to become as aerobically fit as possible, given the constraints of your busy, hectic life; and you need to do strengthening and mobility exercises.

We need to use the calculator, but we need to use it intelligently. I want you to run your 5k, take off 5-10 seconds, plug that performance into the calculator and see what performance you get for the marathon. This will be the goal performance for the time being. After you have run some predictor workouts, such as the Yasso 800s, and some marathon-pace workouts, you will get a better sense of what you can run on race day.

One final and important thing to mention about the 5k race: the best 5k races are run with even splits through the first 3 miles (roughly 4,800m), and finish with a fast 200m *kick* (which is just a term for running fast at the end of a race). This is called a negative split race, with the last half of the race being faster than the first half of the race. If you haven't run a 5k in weeks or months, then you might struggle to execute a negative split race. Most runners will run a positive split race, running the first half of the race faster than the second half of the race. No one wants to endure the pain of going out too hard in a race, then suffering for the last mile or more of the race. With this in mind, I suggest you run the first mile very conservatively. You need to run a pace that is challenging, yet comfortable for the first half mile. People will pass you and that's to be expected since 80-90% of people in the race will run a positive split race. Don't be one of these people. We need an accurate measure of your fitness, and the best way to get this is for you to execute a negative split race.

Okay, enough about the 5k at the end of the week. Here is what the week looks like leading up to the race: Monday is the same as the three previous weeks, but Friday will be a pre-race day, which I will explain shortly. The Tuesday workout is a fartlek workout. It will be challenging because you switch from 3 minutes *on*, 2 minutes *steady*, to 4 minutes *on*, to 1 minute *steady* during the workout. Four minutes *on*, with 1 minute *steady*, is both a physical and mental challenge, but you're ready to do this workout – the most difficult workout yet. This is a continuous run, 60 minutes total with the warm-up and cool-down. SAM Hard will be challenging again this week, even though you've done the routine twice at this point. Don't worry about the SAM Hard impacting your ability to race on Saturday. Your legs will be recovered by

Saturday. And remember, we're training through the race on Saturday.

Wednesday's run can be bumped up 5 minutes from the week before, and this may be a run where you feel a bit flat. This run will not be in your legs on Saturday, and you will get a nice aerobic stimulus by running 65 minutes. Go straight into SAM Easy for a stimulus that is close to 75 minutes. As always, if you are tired at the 40 or 45 minute mark of the Wednesday run, simply run 60 minutes and feel good about your day (but still do SAM Easy at the end of the run).

Thursday is only 45 minutes of cross training. You're not gaining fitness on Thursday, but maintaining fitness, and it will help your legs feel fresh for Saturday's 5k.

Friday is your first pre-race day. The pre-race is the same for all races. The concept here is simple. You need to run a bit to warm up and do some strides at 5k pace so that the pace of the race feels comfortable the next day. Do LMLS to start, then run 10 or 15 minutes of easy jogging to warm-up, do 5 x 20 second strides with 60-90 seconds of easy jogging, and cool down 10 minutes. Do the mobility exercises from Phase 1 SAM Easy to finish the pre-race day. Please don't run more than assigned, and please don't run faster than 5k pace on pre-race day.

If you were focused on the 5k as your primary race distance, then you would do some strides faster than 5k pace on pre-race day. However, 5k is not your primary distance, marathon distance is, so this is certainly not the day to challenge yourself to run faster than 5k pace.

Saturday is pretty simple. Do the pre-race warm-up that you did on Friday. You're going to do LMLS, a 10-15 minute easy jog, then 4-5 x 20 second strides (with 60-90 seconds recovery). You want to finish your last stride roughly 1-2 minutes before the start of the race. Now it's time to execute a great race!

Following the race, jog 10 minutes to cool down and then do SAM Easy. You need to try to do the SAM work at the race, but the worst case scenario is that you do it at home. If this is the case, then please do leg swings from LMLS before you get into the car. At some point in the afternoon or evening you need to get in the AIF rope stretching to help lengthen muscles that were shortened during the race.

Sunday is a shorter walk, but you need to keep the pace brisk. You don't need more than 35 to 60 minutes of walking to recover from the race, but you do need to walk briskly to get good blood flow to your lower extremities.

You've now ended the first phase of the 20-week marathon training cycle! You've built good aerobic fitness and you've gained muscular strength. You'll continue to build both of these elements in the coming weeks, but you should take a moment to look back on these first four weeks and feel good about what you've accomplished. Marathon training isn't a walk in the park, but if you're patient and consistent in your training you'll run a great marathon on race day.

TRAINING WEEKS 5-8:

LEARNING TO WORK THE SYSTEM

—— ——

"Real change happens on the level of
the gesture. One person doing one thing
differently than he or she has done before."

— Cheryl Strayed

CHAPTER 7

Week 5

Week Five is an easy recovery week, until you get to Saturday, when the assignment is 13 miles, the longest run you've done so far in the SMT system.

Rest and recovery are key components of all sound running training. In the SMT system you must recover from races. Most people are accustomed to taking a day or two easy after their race, but that's it. You need the week to start with recovery days so that you don't run the risk of getting injured following last week's race. Post-race injuries often come from running when you have asymmetric soreness or pain. For instance, if your left hamstring is tight, the body adjusts in numerous ways to compensate, which often leads to injuries on the opposite side of the body. The SMT system gives you a great chance to stay injury-free because the system has recovery days assigned after races. Your job is to trust the system and trust that you are better off taking a couple of easy days of rest now, rather than having to take a couple of days off later in the training cycle due to a minor injury.

WEEK 5

M   Day off - no running or cross training. If you must do something you can do the mobility work from SAM and you can do rope stretching.

T   LMLS, 60 minutes easy cross training, SAM Easy.

W   LMLS, 45 minutes easy, SAM Easy.

Th   LMLS, 45-55 minutes easy cross training, SAM Easy.

F   LMLS, 45 minutes easy with 5 x 20 second strides (60-90 seconds easy recovery), SAM Easy.

S   LMLS, 13 miles easy, then immediately into SAM Hard.

Su   Brisk walk of 60 to 75 minutes, LMLS before and SAM Easy afterward is encouraged.

On Monday following the race you might be surprised that you are taking a complete day off from running. You never want to take the first day after the race to be sedentary, for the reasons we covered previously. Getting blood flow to damaged muscle tissue and taking inventory of how your body feels post-race are key aspects of the recovery process. The Sunday brisk walk is designed for just this occasion, so Monday—48 hours post race—is the day to take off.

Tuesday is a cross training day of 45 minutes. You need to keep this day easy; between LMLS and SAM you'll get a 60-minute stimulus. On Wednesday you will go for a 45-minute easy run. No strides, but rather a day where you see how everything feels. If there is soreness or pain in a specific place then you need to have the courage to stop the run. Ninety-five percent of runners won't have any issues and will be able to enjoy a nice, easy run. That said, you won't know if you are 100% healthy until you are running, so be cautious and run a short route or run on the treadmill so that you can stop early if need be. Starting on Thursday you are back to a normal schedule. Cross training on Thursday, followed by an easy run with strides on Friday. These two days set you up for a good Saturday long run.

Saturday's long run is 13 miles. There is no reason to speed up at the end of this run. Just get the time in on your feet and finish saying, "I could have run another mile at that pace." The next day you need to walk briskly for 60 minutes, 15 minutes longer than the walks in the previous weeks. The brisk walk is a great way to end the first five weeks of training. By this point, you've learned the rhythm of the week, you've gained both aerobic fitness and muscular strength, you've raced a 5k to determine a baseline fitness, and you've recovered from the 5k race. Now you are ready to handle more running volume and more intensity. Week Six has a challenging workout that you will do three times in the 20-week marathon cycle: Yasso 800s.

Week 6

This week you will do your first Yasso 800s workout, a challenging workout that is a key component in the SMT system as it provides a fairly accurate estimate of marathon fitness. This method has tried and tested results in helping to reasonably predict a goal finishing time for the marathon. The long run increases by 1 mile to a 14-mile run. When you combine a challenging workout on Tuesday with your longest run to date, Week Six is definitely the most challenging thus far. Also, note that the strides are now 25 seconds in duration, rather than the 20-second strides you've done up to this point.

Week Six is the first week of training where both the workout and the long run are quite challenging. This week you will need to bring a sharp focus to both the Tuesday workout and the Saturday long run, as you will be tested much earlier in the workout and long run than you have previously been accustomed to.

Note: Strides are now 25 seconds per stride.

M   LMLS, 50 minutes easy with 5 x 25 second strides (60-90 seconds easy recovery), SAM Easy.

T   Pre-race warm-up, Yasso 800s - 8 x 800m with 400m jog, 10-minute cool-down jog, then SAM Hard.

W   LMLS, 60 minutes easy, SAM Easy.

Th   LMLS, 45-60 minutes easy cross training, SAM Easy.

F   LMLS, 45-50 minutes easy with 5 x 25 second strides (60-90 seconds easy recovery), SAM Easy.

S   LMLS, 14 miles easy, then immediately into SAM Hard.

Su   Brisk walk of 60 to 80 minutes, LMLS before and SAM Easy afterward is encouraged.

WEEK 6

Monday you will run 50 minutes, just as you've been doing for the past few weeks. The one change to Monday is that you need to run 25-second strides rather than the 20-second strides you have been running up to this point. You're ready for this subtle increase, so no need to worry.

Tuesday's workout is one that you may have heard of or perhaps done in your training for previous marathons: Yasso 800s. I love this workout because it's simple. Simplicity is a good thing in workouts where the last 10-20% of the workout is extremely challenging. All you do is run an 800m repetition (two laps around the track), then jog for 400m (one lap around the track). You continue doing this until you've completed eight 800s. That's the workout, nice and simple. What I love about the workout is that by the time you get to the final two 800s, you're in tune with the workout and can push the pace as hard as your fitness will allow.

Yasso 800s are named after their creator, Bart Yasso. In addition to the workout being simple, the workout has a predictive quality for marathon runners. Bart, through his own training and trial and error, found that when he could do ten 800m repetitions and average, for instance, 3 minutes and 40 seconds, he could run a marathon in 3 hours and 40 minutes. Bart's marathon PR is 2:42:26.

Obviously you need to know what he did for the recovery, and this is straightforward. The recovery is 400m and it should be run in the same time it takes you to run the 800m. Here's an example: Let's say you can run 3 minutes and 30 seconds for eight 800s, jogging 400m at roughly 3 minutes and 30 seconds as your recovery. You can use this workout as a rough predictor of marathon performance. Take the time you ran the 800s (3 minutes and 30 seconds), add 5 seconds. In this example you should be able to run a marathon in 3 hours and 35 minutes.

You will start with eight Yasso 800s this week and will build up to ten 800s in Week Fourteen. There are several subtleties with this workout, both in the execution and its predictive nature. This workout, as with all of the other workouts you will do in the SMT system, needs to be done with negative splits. When you're doing eight 800s, shoot for six at about the same pace, then faster on number seven, and fastest on number eight. Unlike the other workouts in the SMT system, you should run close to a race effort in this workout. You need to end the workout saying, "If I had an 800m jog rather than a 400m jog I probably could have done one more, but I'm so glad this workout is over." This workout is just one notch below race effort, whereas most other workouts in the SMT system are a couple notches below race effort.

I've had many athletes use Yasso 800s in their training and there are two things to keep in mind when using the workout as a predictor of marathon performance. The first is that the workout is an accurate predictor of marathon performance if, and only if, the athlete does several long runs of 18 miles or longer. Second, the athlete needs to have decent running volume throughout the training cycle. The SMT system follows the *Goldilocks* principle: the volume you're running in the five days per week that you run is not too much and not too little, it is *just right*, letting your body recover and allowing you to stay on top of all the other obligations in your life.

If you run the Tuesday workouts, the Wednesday *tired legs runs* and the Saturday long runs, you'll get in the requisite volume needed to run a good marathon. The flip side is, many runners will do Yasso 800s and assume they can run a marathon at the pace predicted by the Yasso workout, yet these athletes don't run a significant long run each week and aren't running enough volume during the week to run the predicted marathon finishing time. The most common result for these runners is that they can run the predicted marathon race pace for 20 miles, but slow down significantly (sometimes as much as a minute per mile) in the final 6.2 miles of the marathon. Don't let this happen to you! Embrace the SMT system, work the SMT system, and you'll run the great marathon that you're capable of.

The final aspect of Yasso 800s that you need to understand is that many runners find that the workout predicts a time that is approximately 5 minutes faster than they can actually run. In our example of the runner who can run 3:30 for ten 800s, this means that they should plan to run their marathon at approximately 3:35 pace. But remember, this rule of thumb is coming from a large cross section of runners, many of whom are not doing four 18-mile runs, two 20-mile runs, and one 22-mile run in the SMT 20-week period.

The whole reason you're doing Yasso 800s is to help you figure out your marathon pace in training. While it's a decent and mostly accurate predictor of your marathon fitness, the reason it is part of the SMT system is that we can get a sense of your marathon pace without having you race a half marathon.

Racing a half marathon in the middle of a marathon cycle is sound (we will discuss this at the end of the book), yet the problem is that it takes close to two weeks to fully recover from the half marathon. By running some Yasso 800 workouts in a marathon cycle you can get in more training with a 20-week cycle. The Yasso 800 workout is difficult, but you will be recovered by Saturday for your long run.

You'll notice that to prepare for this workout you'll do a pre-race warm-up, the same warm-up you did before the 5k race. Nothing complicated, but this is a warm-up that will get you ready to run a faster workout on the track. Most people will start the strides at 5k pace and finish with the last couple of strides faster than 5k pace. You're warming up for the workout, so don't worry if you don't feel snappy in the first couple strides.

Make sure you allow enough time for this workout. Obviously the amount of time for the pre-race warm-up and the 10 minute cool-down jog are set, but the duration of the workout can vary widely. If you are running your 800s in 4 minutes, then plan on roughly 82 minutes for the Yasso 800s portion of the workout; if you are running 3:30 for your 800s, plan on roughly 70 minutes; if your 800s are at 3-minute pace, the Yasso 800s will take you roughly 60 minutes.

Wednesday is only 60 minutes—less than what you are ready to handle, which would be a 70-minute run. Sixty minutes makes much more sense the day following a Yasso 800 workout because you will likely have some soreness in the hamstrings and lower legs, and there is no reason to get greedy with the training. Sixty minutes following a hard workout is a solid two-day block of training, so don't feel like you should have run more than 60 minutes. Friday's assignment is 45-50 minutes easy with strides, which will soon become 55 minutes in the coming weeks.

Saturday's run is simply one more mile than two weeks before: 14 miles. What's noteworthy about this run is that long runs get exponentially more difficult as you add mileage. While the increase from 13 miles to 14 miles is the appropriate step this week, there is a chance that you will feel more fatigue Saturday afternoon than you have up to this point in the training. If you don't feel any more fatigue this Saturday than usual, that's great, but know that you will soon need to plan your future Saturdays to allow for a possible nap in the afternoon. Sunday is the crucial 60-80 minute brisk-walk.

Week 7

Several of the runs will increase by 5 minutes in this week of training. You can definitely handle all of these increases as the next step in a safe and sound training progression. Tuesday looks like a simple workout, but as I've observed before, *simple ain't easy*. Don't expect Tuesday to be easy. Saturday is the first long run where you should try to speed up in the last 3 miles of the run if you feel strong and energetic. If you don't feel strong and energetic on Saturday, just get in the 14 miles and feel good about your day's accomplishment.

WEEK 7

M   LMLS, 55 minutes easy with 5 x 25 second strides (60-90 seconds easy recovery), SAM Easy.

T   LMLS, 10-minute warm-up, 45 minutes of 4 minutes on, 1 minute steady fartlek, 10-minute cool-down, SAM Hard.

W   LMLS, 60-70 minutes easy, SAM Easy.

Th LMLS, 45-60 minutes easy cross training, SAM Easy.

F   LMLS, 55 minutes easy with 5 x 25 second strides (60-90 seconds easy recovery), SAM Easy.

S   LMLS, 14 miles easy and if you feel good, at the 11-mile mark you can speed up a bit in the last 3 miles, then immediately into SAM Hard.

Su Brisk walk of 60 to 85 minutes, LMLS before and SAM Easy afterward is encouraged.

Monday you need to run 55 minutes rather than the 50 minutes you've run in the last few weeks. A 55-minute run will be the normal Monday assignment for the rest of the training cycle.

Tuesday definitely falls into the *simple ain't easy* category of training. Your workout is simply 45 minutes of fartlek, specifically 4 minutes *on*, 1 minute *steady*. This is a challenging workout and you should get to the 35-minute mark of the workout fatigued and looking forward to the end. Stay focused and try to run the last two 4-minute *on* portions faster than you've been running.

Finish the workout saying, "I had one more 4-minute repetition in me, but it would have been a race effort to do two more, and I don't know if I could have done that." SAM Hard will be challenging, but at this point in the training you know how to stay focused during this work. You simply need to get it done.

On Wednesday run 70 minutes if you're feeling strong and energetic, or 60 minutes if you feel average or tired. This is the first run where you will likely experience tired legs in the run. Two reasons for this: the subtle increase in volume of 5 minutes from Week Four (when you ran 65 minutes) and the intensity of Tuesday's workout. During Wednesday's workout, run as slow as you need to run to finish, saying "I could have run 10 or even 15 more minutes." This statement needs to be true for a run that is 70 minutes, but also true for runs that are 90 minutes, which you will do later in the training cycle. Feeling strong and energetic on Wednesday is a great indicator that, as Bob Kennedy said, "You are on top of the training." The final point is Wednesday is a key day in the SMT system marathon cycle, giving you the volume that is necessary to run a good marathon, and giving you the confidence and experience that you can run a solid pace when your legs are tired in the final miles of the marathon.

You'll run 55 minutes on Friday, rather than the 45 or 50 minutes you have been doing. You will stop at 55 minutes for Monday and Friday as the maximum duration for these easy days. While you can make the argument that you could handle more running on these days, there are two reasons not to do more than 55 minutes. The first is that these days take 70 minutes to complete due to the LMLS and SAM. Busy adults usually can't fit in much more than 70 minutes on their easy days due to the hectic pace of life.

Second, while volume is important, the most important days of the week are the Saturday long run and the Tuesday workout. If you were assigned 60, 65, or 70 minutes there is a greater chance that you will enter a Saturday long run or Tuesday workout fatigued from these easy days. Now is a good time to remember one of the cardinal virtues of the SMT system: *keep your easy days easy, so your hard days can be hard*. Specifically, keep Monday and Friday easy so that Tuesday and Saturday can be hard.

Saturday's long run is the first long run where you will need to do a good job of being honest with yourself about how you're feeling in the final miles of the run. The assignment is 14 miles. If you feel good at the 11-mile mark you can speed up a bit in the last 3 miles. Here's the key to the workout: you don't *need* to speed up at this point. While the option

there, having the courage to maintain pace if you're f

on this long run. Today you should keep Coach Vern

forefront of your mind: *need to do* vs. *nice to do*. Runr

to do, but speeding up at the 11-mile mark is the *ni*

good at 11 miles then you have the green light to spee

secondary to getting in the time on your feet and com

Please be honest with yourself when you hit the 1

few moments checking in with your body. If you're fee

the choice right then and there that you won't speed up when you hit the 11-mile point.

If you're feeling strong at 10 miles, say to yourself, "I'll run one more mile and if I still feel good at the 11-mile mark, I'll speed up." Proper self-talk is all-important for running appropriate pace, distance, and possessing positivity. Think of your self-talk as the little coach inside constantly monitoring the athlete who is in need of consistent counsel and encouragement.

The most important mile of the entire week is mile 10 to 11 of the Saturday long run. The phrase "make the right choice" appears throughout the book for a reason, and the reason is to help you maximize the time you spend training. You're going to get a great aerobic stimulus if you complete the 14-mile run, so please don't speed up at 11 miles if you are feeling *poor*. The definition of poor that I'm intending here is "worse than usual." If you make the wrong choice and decide to speed up at mile 11 when you are feeling average or poor, you set yourself up for a possible cycle of overtraining. Overtraining doesn't happen from one hard workout, but from a series of bad choices. If you fail to make the right choice on Saturday, you'll get to Tuesday's workout feeling a bit flat. Next Tuesday's workout is a longer workout (70 minutes) and while you might start the workout feeling energetic and fresh, there is a good chance you won't be able to finish the workout strong as you will still be feeling the effects of the long run.

The SMT system has more days built in between the hard days to prevent this from happening (e.g., you have a brisk walk on Sunday and an easy day on Monday to recover from Saturday's long run) but the system works optimally when you make the right choices throughout the training. Bottom line: make the right choice on the long run this week.

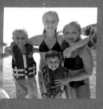

py New Year
ie Schoening

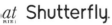

Merriest
CHRISTMAS

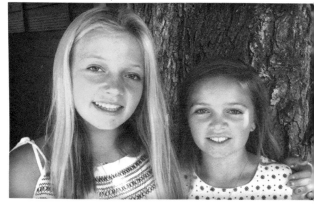

The brisk walk on Sunday may not feel good in the first 30 minutes, but you'll likely feel good by the end of the walk. Please don't cut these walks short. You need to get in at least 60 minutes.

Week 8

There are two big aerobic challenges this week. A progression run on Tuesday and a big jump in long run mileage on Saturday: a 16-mile long run. Between these two runs is a Wednesday run where you have the option of running up to 75 minutes. Seventy-five minutes is where the Wednesday run can start to feel like a long-ish run. Please, make the right choice and only run 75 minutes on Wednesday if you're feeling great. Otherwise, run 60 minutes on Wednesday and feel good about your training day. Finally, make sure you are mentally ready on Saturday to not only run the 16-mile run but also to be ready to do some solid SAM Hard work following the run. Saturday will be your hardest training day to date and you need to be ready to handle both the run and the SAM Hard work.

M	LMLS, 55 minutes easy with 5 x 25 second strides (60-90 seconds easy recovery), SAM Easy.
T	LMLS, 10-minute warm-up, 50 minute progression run: 20 minutes steady, 15 minutes faster, 10 minutes faster, 5 minutes fastest but controlled, 10-minute cool-down, SAM Hard.
W	LMLS, 60-75 minutes easy, SAM Easy.
Th	LMLS, 45-60 minutes easy cross training, SAM Easy.
F	LMLS, 55 minutes easy with 5 x 25 second strides (60-90 seconds easy recovery), SAM Easy.
S	LMLS, 16 miles easy, then immediately into SAM Hard.
Su	Brisk walk of 60-90 minutes, LMLS before and SAM Easy afterward is encouraged.

WEEK 8

The progression run on Tuesday is another workout that falls into the *simple ain't easy* category. The progression is 20 minutes steady, 15 minutes faster, 10 minutes faster, 5 minutes fastest, but controlled. As with all of the progression runs, you should be able to finish saying you could have run 5 to 10 more minutes at the final pace.

Be conservative with the initial 20-minute portion. You must be able to change pace three times in this workout and you need to be able to change gears mentally when you are tired. To get the body to change pace and speed up, the mind must make a choice to run faster. Obviously, this doesn't always work and there are times when you ask your body to speed up and it can't. The point here is that you need to practice making a choice to change paces and have your body respond to this request.

As with all progression runs, you need to finish running controlled. What is controlled? Controlled is knowing you could have run 5 more minutes at the final pace. This is not a race effort and you should not be going all-out. Stay focused at the end of the running part of the workout so that you are ready for a rigorous SAM Hard session. You'll get a great 85 to 90 minute stimulus by going directly from 70 minutes of running to 15 to 20 minutes of SAM work. You may be on Phase 2 of the SAM progression or you may be on Phase 3 or 4 of the SAM progression. Regardless, stay focused and bring as much energy as you can to this part of the workout.

Wednesday is 60-75 of minutes easy running. I recommend you shoot for 70 minutes, and if you feel great you can go 5 more minutes. This is how you will treat all of the Wednesday runs moving forward. There will be a minimum volume you need to run and then there will be a longer option that you can run if you are feeling fantastic. Be certain to make the right choice on Wednesday. *When in doubt, do less* and run 60 minutes easy. You had a hard day 24 hours earlier and you're gaining aerobic fitness by getting in the minimum run. Resist the temptation of over-training. You may think you're doing the right thing by stuffing in more but you will likely pay the price of injury and/or incapacitating fatigue. In keeping with less is more, it's crucial in Week Eight to keep Thursday's cross training easy and keep Friday's easy run easy. It's called easy for a reason.

Saturday is a long run of 16 miles, a 2-mile increase from the previous week. In the SMT system there is a simple approach to increasing long run volume. Early in the training, when you need to be cautious with building the long run, increasing a mile each week is responsible. However, once you get to Week Eight in the training, all of the SAM work you've done has given you the muscular strength to handle longer runs. Going from 14 miles to 16 miles is not a reckless jump in mileage, as long as you keep the run easy. The goal is simple: get in 16 miles on your feet, without the assumption that you will speed up in the last few 2-3 miles. At this point in your training, 16 miles is a serious run, and what is important at this juncture in your training is to get time in on your feet, nothing fancy, just point A to point B, however long it takes. Because the SAM work needs to come immediately following the 16-mile run, this will be the most challenging workout to date, so be prepared to be mentally and physically challenged. You may need a nap Saturday afternoon to recover from your longest effort to date.

Week Eight is a big week, and you need to make sure you are resting and recovering throughout the week. When the long runs are 16 miles and longer, fatigue can easily set in. Keep your legs fresh and your energy high by keeping all of the easy days easy. There are four easy days each week and only two hard days, plus "half a hard day" on Wednesday. You have ample opportunity to recover from the training, training which will continue to become greater in both volume and intensity in the coming weeks. As long as you make the right choices each week in terms of food, sleep, and hydration, you'll be able to train at a high level.

TRAINING WEEKS 9-12:

SERIOUS TRAINING PART 1

WELCOME TO THE LONG RUN

"Action may not always bring happiness,
but there is no happiness without action."

— Benjamin Disraeli

CHAPTER 8

Week 9

As you can probably guess, both Tuesday and Saturday will be challenging days. The Tuesday workout looks similar to the workout you did in Week Three, but it presents a formidable challenge as you'll be doing one more 8-minute repetition. I'll explain below, but the bottom line is: Be ready for a challenging workout! The long run is 16 miles, just like last week, but this week you should speed up in the last 3 miles of the run if you're feeling up to it. Again, just getting in the 16 miles is the first goal on Saturday, but there is a very good chance you will be feeling strong, in which case you can speed up. Wednesday gives you the option of running 80 minutes (5 minutes longer than last week) if you're feeling in fine fettle. Finally, strides on Monday and Friday are now 30 seconds long. Thirty seconds is the longest stride you will do in the 20-week training cycle.

Note: Strides are now 30 seconds per stride.

M   LMLS, 55 minutes easy with 5 x 30 second strides (60-90 seconds easy recovery), SAM Easy.

T   LMLS, 10-minute warm-up, 5 x 8 minutes at a challenging pace with 3-minute steady recoveries, 10-minute cool-down, SAM Hard.

W   LMLS, 60-80 minutes easy, SAM Easy.

Th   LMLS, 45-60 minutes easy cross training, SAM Easy.

F   LMLS, 55 minutes easy with 5 x 30 second strides (60-90 seconds easy recovery), SAM Easy.

S   LMLS, 16 miles easy and if you feel good, at the 13-mile mark you can speed up a bit in the last 3 miles, then immediately into SAM Hard.

Su   Brisk walk of 60-85 minutes, LMLS before and SAM Easy afterward is encouraged.

WEEK 9

Before we go on I need to discuss the SAM work, now that you've done this work for eight weeks. The SAM work is obviously a huge component of the SMT system. I want to be clear that there is nothing wrong with being at Phase 2 or Phase 3 SAM work at this point. That said, this is Week Nine and it means you may have moved through Phase 4 of the SAM progression. For the upcoming weeks, take note of the following guidelines.

First, if SAM has been a challenge and you're not able to efficiently move through the exercises in the Phase 4 SAM routines, then simply stay at your current level until you feel ready to progress. From now until Week Eighteen, the running portion of the training is extremely challenging, so if your SAM work is at Phase 2 or Phase 3, don't feel bad about simply maintaining that level of work for the remainder of the training cycle. That said, you may feel strong and like you can definitely do Phase 4, perhaps even move to Phase 5 of SAM training. If so, that's great. But once you get to Week Thirteen of the training then you will simply maintain the SAM work that you're doing. You don't need to advance to the next phase of SAM work from Week Thirteen on.

Phase 5 is the final phase of SAM work for this marathon training cycle. After you go through the 20-week SMT cycle successfully, you may add some more intense SAM work—such as kettlebell exercises—to your training for your second 20-week marathon cycle. For the first 20-week cycle, simply trust that Phase 5 SAM is a solid amount of work to be doing.

The final aspect of SAM work that you need to understand is that from here on out, SAM will take more time as you move through the progression of phases. SAM Hard days will go from roughly 15 minutes of work to 20-25 minutes of work. Carve out an additional 10 minutes in your day. I know it may seem like you don't have 10 more minutes in your day, but these 10 minutes are going to make a terrific impact on your fitness. Find these 10 minutes! They will make you a better runner and they will result in a better marathon performance.

This week's Tuesday workout is slightly longer than you've done before, with 72 minutes of running as the assignment. When you factor in LMLS and SAM, it puts you at 90 minutes start to finish, so make sure you have enough time carved out of your day to get this workout done. The workout is the same workout you did in Week Three, only this time, add one more 8-minute repetition. You need to keep the steady portions steady; running slowly on the 3-minute portions is not the intent of this workout. You need to finish this workout saying you could have done at least one more 8-minute repetition and it would not have been at race effort. Unlike many of the workouts you do in the

SMT system, you don't have to say, "I could have done two more repetitions." 8 minutes is a long repetition and you should be running fast enough on each repetition in this workout that doing seven repetitions would be out of the question.

Wednesday is 60-80 minutes. You need to embrace the idea that a slow 60-minute run is fine today. That said, the workout on Tuesday wasn't a killer workout, so there is a good chance that you will want to run 80 minutes. Today is one of the first really important days to "make the right choice." If you are feeling flat and a bit tired, but decide you need to run 80 minutes to feel good about yourself, that's a bad choice. Alternatively, you might get to the 50-minute mark and say, "I feel good today. I haven't run 80 minutes before on a Wednesday, but today I know I can. This should be fun." Remember, if you choose to run 80 minutes, you should finish the run saying, "I could have gone 90 minutes, but it would have been a challenge." Bottom line: you need to make the right choice today so you can rock your long run on Saturday.

This week's 16-mile long run is the most important day of the week. Goal number one is to get in the 16 miles. You need to get in this distance so that you can keep progressing the duration of the long run. If you feel good at the 13-mile mark, speed up a bit. There is a good chance you will feel like speeding up at 13 miles. If you get to this point in the run and you feel average or poor, just get in the 16 miles and feel good about your accomplishment.

16 miles is a significantly different long run than the first long run of this training cycle, which was 10 miles. 16 miles is an important distance in the SMT system because it's a distance that begins teaching you how to run well when you're fatigued. Simply put, long runs shorter than 16 miles don't pose this type of challenge for a fit runner, but even fit runners have to focus in the final miles of the 16-mile run to keep from slowing down. This means that not only is this run a great aerobic stimulus, it's also a great psychological stimulus.

Finish the week with a brisk walk. If you can do the 90-minute walks, do so, as each minute walking is like money in the bank. There will certainly be more than one Sunday when you are pressed to make any time at all to walk, much less the full 90 minutes. Make every effort to fit in at least 30 minutes of brisk walking each Sunday. You shouldn't do just 30 minutes of brisk walking week in and week out, but it's understandable that you may need to do so a couple times over a 20-week cycle. That said, you must do something on Sundays to get good blood flow to the legs. If you are sedentary the day after a long run, you set yourself up for a more difficult training week on Monday.

Week 10

This is a straightforward yet demanding week. Yasso 800s on Tuesday and then your first 18-mile run on Saturday. This week you will do nine 800s in the Yasso workout, one more than last time. Because you need to run hard—running to 97% of your capabilities in the Yasso workout—Wednesday is a slightly easier run. As strenuous as the Tuesday Yasso workout is, Saturday presents an even greater challenge. The 18-mile run is much more difficult than a 16-mile run, and for this reason you need to be rested and ready for a great run come Saturday. Obviously the SAM Hard assignment following the run will be the most difficult SAM Hard you've done up to this point. Trust that you're ready to handle all that this week brings.

WEEK 10

M   LMLS, 55 minutes easy with 5 x 30 second strides (60-90 seconds easy recovery), SAM Easy.

T   Pre-race warm-up, Yasso 800s - 9 x 800m with 400m jog, 10-minute cool-down jog, then SAM Hard.

W   LMLS, 60-70 minutes easy, SAM Easy.

Th LMLS, 45-60 minutes easy cross training, SAM Easy.

F   LMLS, 55 minutes easy with 5 x 30 second strides (60-90 seconds easy recovery), SAM Easy.

S   LMLS, 18 miles easy then immediately into SAM Hard after the run.

Su Brisk walk of 60-85 minutes, LMLS before and SAM Easy afterward is encouraged.

In my experience, roughly half of runners execute their first Yasso 800s workout correctly, running consistent times for the first six, faster on seven and eight, with the fastest repetition on number nine. This execution of the workout is absolutely fine and to be expected. That said, this week you should take the average 800m split from the workout in Week Six and use that to guide you for the first six of the nine 800s you will be running in this workout. Feel free to start a few seconds slower on reps one and two than you averaged in Week Six. These longer repetitions often take time to feel comfortable and you can make up the time in the middle repetitions.

The goal for today's Yasso workout is to run all nine 800s and run a negative split workout. Simple assignment, but it won't be easy. Just like the last time you ran Yasso 800s, you want to be running just below race effort—so 97% effort—on the ninth repetition. You should be able to say, "I might have been able to do a tenth repetition, but I would have needed 800m to recover. I could not have done a tenth repetition with just 400m recovery." This workout is different than most SMT system workouts for the simple fact that when you finish the workout you have come very close to running as fast as you are capable of. Today you can take roughly 5 minutes following the workout before you go into SAM Hard, yet you must focus on SAM Hard and get through the routines energetically. This is great training for your brain.

You'll be extremely tired following the 800s, but asking your body to do difficult SAM Hard when you're tired is good training for asking your body to maintain pace in the final 6.2 miles of a marathon. Yes, there is a physical benefit to doing SAM Hard following an extremely challenging workout, but I would argue that following a workout where you are running close to all out, SAM Hard is strengthening your will for the unique challenge of racing a marathon. And this, dear athletes, is our raison d'être.

You will get a bit of a respite on Wednesday for the simple fact that Tuesday was so demanding. Plan to run just 60 minutes. Only run 70 minutes if you feel great at the 55-minute mark and want to run a bit more.

SMT strikes a balance between hard workouts and long runs on one side, and rest and recovery on the other side. If you run 60 minutes easy on Wednesday, cross train easy for 60 minutes on Thursday, and run your normal Friday run with strides, you will be ready for the 18-mile assignment on Saturday. However, you will only be ready to run 18 miles well if you take

Wednesday, Thursday, and Friday easy. You must make the right choices and keep all three of these days relaxed if you want to run well on Saturday.

Saturday falls under the *simple ain't easy* heading. Run 18 miles. It's a simple assignment, but not an easy one. You can go as slow as you need to, but you need to cover 18 miles. You have nine weeks of SAM under your belt and you're aerobically fit, so your body can handle the volume. The only thing that remains is for you to mentally focus for the entire 18-mile distance. It's such a great feeling when you finish the 18 miles on Saturday and have the rest of the weekend to enjoy with friends and loved ones. But remember, you're not finished until you've finished SAM Hard. As you know, it is crucial to do the SAM work as close to the end of the 18-mile run as possible, as the coupling of the run and the SAM Hard work extends the aerobic stimulus without any additional pounding on your legs.

You'll need a brisk walk on Sunday to recover from the run. 18-mile runs (and longer) are your new reality, which means that the Sunday brisk walk is crucial if you are going to run well the following week.

Week 11

This week you'll not only run 18 miles, you also have the green light to speed up the last 3 miles if you're feeling up to it. Eighteen miles is a great run in itself, and when you add the option of speeding up at the end, you have a very tough run. You also have a demanding 50 minute progression run on Tuesday. Because you did a progression run three weeks ago, you know how to execute the workout and should be able to run well on Tuesday. Wednesday you can run as long as 85 minutes, but again, only if you feel well. If you do feel well and run strong on Wednesday, it is a very good indication that you're handling the training. If you're consistently feeling strong on Wednesdays, we know that you are on top of your training.

M   LMLS, 55 minutes easy with 5 x 30 second strides (60-90 seconds easy recovery), SAM Easy.

T   LMLS, 10-minute warm-up, 50 minute progression run: 20 minutes steady, 15 minutes faster, 10 minutes faster, 5 minutes fastest but controlled, 10-minute cool-down, SAM Hard.

W   LMLS, 60-85 minutes easy, SAM Easy.

Th   LMLS, 45-60 minutes easy cross training, SAM Easy.

F   LMLS, 55 minutes easy with 5 x 30 second strides (60-90 seconds easy recovery), SAM Easy.

S   LMLS, 18 miles easy and if you feel good, at the 15-mile mark you can speed up a bit in the last 3 miles, then immediately into SAM Hard.

Su   Brisk walk of 60-90 minutes, LMLS before and SAM Easy afterward is encouraged.

WEEK 11

Tuesday is a progression run. The key to this workout is that you start the run at a conservative pace. You will have to speed up three times in this progression, so set yourself up for a successful workout by being conservative with the steady running pace to start. As with all progression runs, finish saying, "I could have run 5 or 10 more minutes at the final pace." Challenge yourself on Tuesday, but don't make it the hardest workout to date.

Wednesday's assignment is 60-85 minutes. The first goal is to get in 60 minutes, so if you feel flat at the 40-minute mark of this run, then make 60 minutes easy your goal. If you feel good at 60 minutes you can aim for the 85-minute goal. As with all Wednesdays, the first goal is to get in 60 minutes. Do this and you have a solid Tuesday/Wednesday training session. It's all about linking the training days and creating synergy. The whole is greater than the sum of its parts.

Because Tuesday and Wednesday were challenging, you need to make sure that Thursday and Friday are truly easy days. As I said before, SMT training works because there is enough recovery between the hard days, so long as you keep the easy days easy! This week you only have Thursday and Friday to recover in preparation for Saturday.

The number one goal of Saturday is to get in 18 miles. Eighteen miles is a solid run, the longest distance run in many marathon training programs. While you will run 20 and 22 miles in the SMT system, know that 18 miles is a serious run for serious runners. If you feel well at the 15-mile mark then you can run the last 3 miles a bit faster. The pace increase is much less important than getting in 18 miles. Eighteen miles, going as slow as you need to go to cover the distance, is the primary assignment for the day.

SAM Hard immediately following the 18-mile long run is vital. This is a difficult mental and physical challenge, just as running a marathon is a difficult mental and physical challenge. As I've mentioned time and again, doing SAM immediately following the long run is a *need to do,* not *a nice to do* in the SMT system. Prepare your mind to run well in the final miles of the 18-mile run, then go right into SAM.

Sunday's brisk walk is, as always, critical. Week Twelve is going to be even more challenging than Week Eleven and you need to be ready for a dynamic week of training.

Week 12

Steel yourself! Week Twelve is difficult. The workout on Tuesday is hard because you have short rests between the 8-minute repetitions, making the intensity of the workout as high as any you've done up to this point. Saturday is your first 20-mile run. You're ready to run 20 miles, but 20 miles is a different animal than 18 miles, so you'll need to be ready both mentally and physically for the challenge. The Wednesday run moves up by 5 minutes to 90 minutes, the longest that you'll have assigned during the 20-week training cycle.

M LMLS, 55 minutes easy with 5 x 30 second strides (60-90 seconds easy recovery), SAM Easy.

T LMLS, 10-minute warm-up, 5 x 8 minutes at a challenging pace with 2-minute slow recoveries, 10-minute cool-down, SAM Hard.

W LMLS, 60-90 minutes easy, SAM Easy.

Th LMLS, 45-60 minutes easy cross training, SAM Easy.

F LMLS, 50 minutes easy with 5 x 30 second strides (60-90 seconds easy recovery), SAM Easy.

S LMLS, 20 miles easy then immediately into SAM Hard after the run.

Su Brisk walk of 60-90 minutes, LMLS before and SAM Easy afterward is encouraged.

At first glance Tuesday may look like a similar workout to the workout in Week Nine. It's not. The workout in Week Nine had you running 3 minutes steady between the 8-minute segments, making it similar to a fartlek workout. This week you will run 5 x 8 minutes with 2 minutes *slow* between the 8-minute repetitions. Because you're running slowly between the 8-minute repetitions, you can run the 8 minutes much faster than you did in Week Nine. These are aerobic repeats, meaning that the majority of the workout is fueled by the aerobic system. This will be a challenging workout, short but intense. You should finish saying, "I know I could have done one more 8-minute repetition, but I also know I couldn't have done two more." Again, it's a hard workout. SAM Hard will be a mental challenge today, but you can definitely get through the assignment. Take SAM Hard one exercise at a time. Couple the 5 x 8 minutes with 2 minutes slow, followed by SAM Hard, and you'll have had a tremendous day of training.

Think of Wednesday as a release valve in your training. On Tuesday you did a hard workout, and in the previous two weeks you have done your first two 18-mile runs of the training cycle. Are you tired? If the answer is yes, then just run 60 minutes easy and hang 'em up for the day.

If you wake up Wednesday feeling rested, and hit the 45-minute mark of the run feeling strong, you can run longer than 60 minutes. Double-check to make certain you feel good before opting for the extension. This is one of those places in the training where you need to make the right choice. You just did a tough workout on Tuesday and you have your first 20-mile run on Saturday. These are by far the most important days of the week. A 70, 80, or 90-minute Wednesday run is a *nice to do,* not *a need to do.* If you feel great, run 70, 80, or 90 minutes, but if you feel average or a bit fatigued, then just run 60 minutes and start the recovery process, readying yourself for Saturday. Regardless of how far you run on Wednesday, do not speed up at the end of this run. In preparation for Saturday you will run just 50 minutes on Friday.

You need to plan out the 20-mile run before you wake up on Saturday. You need to have your route planned, your hydration set, and your fueling food and drink ready.

You also need to have the option of taking a nap in the afternoon. This is not a Saturday where you run in the morning and then plan a full day of activities following the run. You're going to be fatigued following this run. This is a crucial training run in the SMT system and you need to set up your day for both a successful run and for proper recovery after the run.

GEEK OUT
Read more about The Science of Optimizing Fueling During the Marathon on page 197

When choosing a loop, some runners like to find a 5-mile loop and set their drinks out on a car roof or picnic table, allowing them to quickly run by and get some water or sports drink. I also like the idea of an 18-mile run, then add on 2 miles at the end. Why? Because if for some reason the run is going badly you can opt out at 18. The last 2 miles of a 20-mile run can be exponentially hard on the body if you're having a bad day. A bad 20-mile run will mean that you will likely need to skip Tuesday's workout and resume normal training on Wednesday. A bad 18-mile run is a distance that you can recover from and still do most of Tuesday's workout. I don't mean to scare you; not only are you ready to run 20 miles at this point in the training, you're ready to run it well! I just want you to be aware that if you have that one-in-ten experience of a bad run on Saturday, it's a tough run to recover from, so be shrewd in your training choices.

Obviously SAM Hard following this run will likely be the toughest post-run work you've done in SMT. Please be mentally ready to energetically move through the SAM Hard routines. It's good to have an attack mindset with SAM. Think about it this way: you will be doing SAM Hard at a time that corresponds to the 22- or 23-mile mark in your marathon. You have to be extremely tough and focused at this juncture in a marathon, and SAM Hard at the end of today's 20-mile run helps you practice the toughened mindset that will see you through the end of the marathon when you are grinding it out. This is your biggest day of training thus far. You're ready for it—now you just have to execute it.

Sunday's assignment is shorter than normal but non-negotiable, giving you more time with loved ones and friends, since you were training longer on Saturday. Keep the walk brisk, as you only need 45-75 minutes of walking.

Provided all is going well, you should be feeling very good about your fitness. You're ready for the next four weeks of training, which is the most challenging block of training in the 20-week training cycle. You can do it.

TRAINING WEEKS 13-16:

SERIOUS TRAINING
PART 2
___   ___
THE MOST CHALLENGING FOUR WEEKS OF THE TRAINING CYCLE

"Enthusiasm is one of the most powerful engines of success. When you do a thing, do it with all your might. Put your whole soul into it. Stamp it with your own personality. Be active, be energetic, be enthusiastic and faithful, and you will accomplish your object. Nothing great was ever achieved without enthusiasm."

— Ralph Waldo Emerson

CHAPTER 9

Week 13

Tuesday is a progression run, but it's much more challenging than previous progression runs because you'll be running for 60 minutes (plus the 10-minute warm-up and cool-down, so 80 minutes of total running). Following this run you will need to be mentally focused to knock out the SAM Hard work. Saturday is a run that most of my clients really enjoy. It's 18 miles with the last 4 miles a bit faster, so long as you feel strong and energetic. Because you did 20 miles the week before, 18 miles, while challenging, is a distance that you can manage, and hopefully you can increase the pace of the last 4 miles. Wednesday you can run as long as 90 minutes, but there is no reason to do so if you're not feeling great. Make the right choice on Wednesday.

M   LMLS, 55 minutes easy with 5 x 30 second strides (60-90 seconds easy recovery), SAM Easy.

T   LMLS, 10-minute warm-up, 60 minute progression run: 30 minutes steady, 15 minutes faster, 10 minutes faster, 5 minutes fastest but controlled, 10-minute cool-down, SAM Hard.

W   LMLS, 60-90 minutes easy, SAM Easy.

Th   LMLS, 45-60 minutes of easy cross training, SAM Easy.

F   LMLS, 55 minutes easy with 5 x 30 second strides (60-90 seconds easy recovery), SAM Easy.

S   LMLS, 18 miles easy and if you feel good, at the 14-mile mark you can speed up a bit in the last 4 miles, then immediately into SAM Hard.

Su   Brisk walk of 60-90 minutes, LMLS before and SAM Easy afterward is encouraged.

WEEK 13

Tuesday's workout that is formidable, but not so much so that you should be intimidated. Tuesday is 80 minutes of total running, with a 60-minute progression run in the middle. Two weeks ago you ran a 50-minute progression run. The difference today is that you run these additional 10 minutes at the start of the progression, which means you are running 30 minutes steady before you have to speed up. You need to be ready to speed up three times during the workout, which is simple on paper but not easy to do in the middle of a progression run. You're ready to do this, and the workout will go well as long as you start the 30-minute steady portion conservatively. This is a great workout mentally because speeding up in the middle of a progression run takes focus, and for this reason, progression runs have a prominent place in the SMT system. Final thought: as with all progression runs, you need to be able to say, "I could have continued the last pace for 5 more minutes, and perhaps 10 minutes, but that likely would have been a race effort."

While Tuesday was not easy, it shouldn't have been a killer day and therefore Wednesday can be a longer run. Sixty to 90 minutes is the assignment. You no doubt know what to do today. The first goal is 60 minutes easy. If you feel good at the 45-minute mark, you can run as many as 90 minutes. Or, you could choose to run 70 or 80 minutes. Choose one of these three options if you feel good and make the choice 45 minutes into the run. Why? If you aren't decisive about the distance you're going to run, the ambitious part of you (ego) will tell you to run longer, yet this may not be the right choice for the day. Make the right choice today.

It's important to note that going right into the SAM Easy after a longish run is another wonderful opportunity to get a long aerobic stimulus. The SAM work will only take you 10 to 15 minutes, but this 10 to 15 minutes is noteworthy when it increases the total workout time to between 70 and 105 minutes (depending on how far you run and how long the SAM Easy work takes you).

You need to have two good recovery days, Thursday and Friday, but by now you should know how to get in the work on these days without being fatigued for the Saturday long run.

Completing 18 miles is far and away the most important goal for Saturday. If you feel great at the 14-mile mark then speed up and run the last 4 miles at a slightly faster pace. At the 11-mile mark, take an honest inventory of how you feel. If you are feeling good, wait until the 14-mile mark and then speed up the last 4 miles. Making the right choice is crucial. Remember, the key for the week is that you get in 18 miles. The 18 mile run is fundamental for running a good marathon and speeding up is a *nice to do,* not *a need to do.* Go into this workout with the mindset of running strong for 18 miles.

You should finish your 18 miles and be able to say, "I definitely could have gone another mile and maintained my pace." Make the right choice today so that you can continue to stay below the threshold of overtraining, as well as staying injury-free. At this point in the SMT system you know that you'll have to be focused to energetically move through the SAM Hard work. Just take this work one exercise at a time and remember that the physical challenge of doing SAM Hard after an 18-mile run is preparing you mentally and physically to run strong in the final miles of the marathon.

Week 14

This is the last week that you will do Yasso 800s. This week, the assignment is ten 800s. A very straight forward assignment, yet also the most difficult workout you've done up to this point (I know, I keep saying this! You're climbing the ladder of fitness). The long run this week is 20 miles, with the goal of speeding up just a bit in the last 3 miles. Simple week, but as you know, *simple ain't easy.*

You need to be rested for the Yasso 800s workout, so if there is any reason that you feel less than 100% when you wake up Tuesday (insert any number of life stresses or sicknesses), then jog easy for 30 minutes on Tuesday and do the workout on Wednesday, resuming Thursday with your regularly scheduled cross training day. You shouldn't run more than 60 minutes on Wednesday as the Yasso workout was very challenging and you need an easier day to recover. The long run is 20 miles this week, and if you feel good, you can speed up the last 3 miles of the run. That said, the number one goal is to simply get in 20 miles on your feet, if you don't feel well at the 17-mile mark, just get to the end of the run, knock out your SAM Hard work and feel very good about your day.

M   LMLS, 55 minutes easy with 5 x 30 second strides (60-90 seconds easy recovery), SAM Easy.

T   Pre-race warm-up, Yasso 800s - 10 x 800m with 400m jog, 10 minute cool-down jog, then SAM Hard.

W   LMLS, 60 minutes easy, SAM Easy.

Th LMLS, 45-60 minutes easy cross training, SAM Easy.

F   LMLS, 50 minutes easy with 5 x 30 second strides (60-90 seconds easy recovery), SAM Easy.

S   LMLS, 20 miles easy and if you feel good, at the 17-mile mark you can speed up a bit in the last 3 miles, then immediately into SAM Hard.

Su Brisk walk of 60-90 minutes, LMLS before and SAM Easy afterward is encouraged.

WEEK 14

The goal for your last Yasso 800s workout is simple: run fast enough that your average for the ten 800s is faster than the previous two workouts. This will not be easy, but given your fitness this is very realistic. The first seven repetitions are to be run at the pace that you've run before in this workout, repetitions eight and nine a bit faster, and on the tenth repetition you need to run at 97%. Don't run all out, but run hard. For today's workout you only need to be able to say this: "If I had another 400m recovery jog then I could have run one more 400m lap at my finishing pace, but no more than that."

You need to be ready to do this workout because it will be used to predict your marathon pace for the upcoming weeks of training. Make sure you get to bed at a good time on Monday so you can execute the workout to the best of your ability.

It's extremely important that you get the average time for your ten 800s. For instance, you might run 800m splits that look like this: 3:40, 3:42, 3:41, 3:41, 3:40, 3:43, 3:40, 3:39, 3:37, 3:34. The average is basically 3:40 for this workout. If you had run a little faster on the workout, say 3:37, then round up to 3:40. If you had run a bit slower than these example splits, for instance an average of 3:43, you still need to round up so that we get a conservative estimate of your fitness. So if you averaged 3:43, use 3:45 as the average 800m split for the workout.

That marathon prediction table in chapter seventeen is very simple. You take your Yasso 800s average 800m split as the starting point. Once you find that number in the table, for instance, 3 minutes and 40 seconds, you see that your corresponding marathon time is 3 hours and 45 minutes. Why the added 5 minutes? You need to add 5 minutes for the correlation between the Yasso workout and your goal marathon time to be an accurate predictor for your goal marathon time. Thousands and thousands of runners have used the Yasso 800m workout to predict their goal marathon time, and for most runners the correlation between the average 800m split and the goal marathon goal time works well, so longs as you tack on 5 minutes to the projected marathon time from the Yasso workout. Now you need to get your goal marathon pace in minutes per mile. In this example we are using 3 hours and 45 minutes as your goal marathon time, which is 8:35 per mile pace; 8:35 is now your marathon pace (MP). You will use MP in the coming weeks in both Tuesday workouts and Saturday long runs.

There is no need for you to do all of this math, so long as you get an average for your 800m splits. Go to the marathon pace table in chapter seventeen to figure out the marathon pace that you'll be running for the remainder of the 20-week training cycle.

Because the Yasso 800m workout is so important in the SMT system, this is a good time to talk about how to tweak your week in the SMT system, sometimes life gets hectic and you aren't going be 100% ready to rock a Yasso 800s workout on Tuesday.

Let's say you have a big day at work on Monday or you had some other life stress that is out of the ordinary. You can move the Tuesday workout back to Wednesday, which is what you should do if you're going to be less than 100% on Tuesday's workout. Do your normal Monday run with strides. Do another run with strides on Tuesday, but run 10 minutes less than you did on Monday. Do these two things and you will be ready to do the Yasso 800s workout on Wednesday.

We've now arrived at the point where athletes make the wrong choice. These athletes *think* they need to get in their normal Wednesday *tired legs run* on Thursday. Wrong! *You don't get to run the Wednesday tired legs run this week!* The SMT system is all about smart training, and smart training puts a high priority on taking training days out when life stress or sickness arise.

Even without *tired legs run*, you've had a great week of training because you got in a hard workout and you'll be able to get in a long run on Saturday (the two most important days). I've had many runners *just* do these two workouts each week and run well, with no Wednesday *tired legs run* in their training schedule ever!

To be clear, if you need to move Tuesday's workout to Wednesday, then you simply resume the training that is written on Thursday, which in this case is 60 minutes of easy cross training.

Remember, making the right choices throughout the 20-week training cycle is the key to your success in the SMT system. Be honest with yourself about your life stress. If you need to move a workout back a day, do so, and feel utterly confident that there is room to make this adjustment.

The Saturday run is your second 20-mile run. You know how to run the distance and you know what you will need to do in the final miles of the run to maintain pace. Many runners will feel good during this run and want to speed up. That's great! If you get to the 17 mile mark feeling strong, you can speed up ever so slightly. Remember, you want to finish this run saying, "I could have run 21 miles today." For this run, you need to respect the distance. As I said earlier, the long run distances get exponentially harder on your body. Twenty miles is a different animal than 18 miles. If you felt great last week and rocked your run, that's great, but be cautious this week. With this in mind, make sure you run your first 10 miles very controlled. Knock out the SAM Hard immediately after the run for your best training day to date. You should feel tremendous satisfaction after the 20 miles and the SAM Hard work. Wow, what a day!

Let me take a moment to describe what would happen if you were to have some life stress pop-up on Friday, making the 20-mile assignment on Saturday unrealistic. The approach is the same as with the Tuesday workout being moved to Wednesday, you will move the Saturday long run to Sunday. When you do this, which is the right choice in this scenario, you can't expect to run well the following Tuesday. Why? Tuesday is 48 hours after your long run on Sunday.

Most athletes *feel a workout* 48 hours afterwards. There is a condition called Delayed Onset Muscle Soreness (DOMS) that simply means that you have the most muscle soreness at some point after you've done a workout. For some people they feel the leg soreness after a long run or workout the next day, but for most recreational runners who are serious about training, DOMS is a 48- hour condition. For this reason, the Tuesday workout needs to be moved to Wednesday.

GEEK OUT
Read more about Delayed Onset Muscle Soreness (DOMS) on page 189

The key here is to accept that making the right choice means moving a long run back a day, to Sunday, and moving a Tuesday workout back a day, to Wednesday. Will you miss a *tired legs run*? Yes. Is this something to worry about? No. Will you, over the course of seven days, get in all of the important workouts you need to continue to improve your aerobic fitness? Yes, as you'll get in a long run (Sunday), a workout (Wednesday), and a long run (Saturday).

Making the right choices when life stress causes your life to go from hectic to chaotic is crucial to your success in the SMT system. Moving a Tuesday workout and moving a Saturday long run are the most common tweaks that need to be made to the training. You can read more about how to tweak the system if and when you get sick and are forced to miss a day of training in

Chapter Thirteen: *The Self-Coached Runner.*

Week 15

This week we are introducing a new type of workout: the marathon pace workout. You will be running marathon pace (MP) for at least part of the Tuesday workouts from now until the race. You're aerobically fit and now you need to prepare yourself to run MP, learning to groove the pace and learning to run marathon pace when you start to feel uncomfortable. Week Fifteen marks another important change in the training. Many of the Tuesday workouts from now to race day will now be assigned as miles. This will likely mean that you have to get up earlier to get in the workout.

WEEK 15

M   LMLS, 55 minutes easy with 5 x 30 second strides (60-90 seconds easy recovery), SAM Easy.

T   LMLS, 2 miles warm-up, 4 miles at MP, 1 mile at HMP, 3 miles at MP, 1 mile cool-down, SAM Hard.

W   LMLS, 60-90 minutes easy, SAM Easy.

Th LMLS, 45-60 minutes easy cross training, SAM Easy.

F   LMLS, 50 minutes easy with 5 x 30 second strides (60-90 seconds easy recovery), SAM Easy.

S   LMLS, 18 miles easy, and if you feel good, run 6 miles at MP from mile 11 to mile 17, finishing with 1 mile easy, then immediately into SAM Hard.

Su Brisk walk of 60-90 minutes, LMLS before and SAM Easy afterward is encouraged.

There is no way around the fact that you have to be running solid volume to be able to run a good marathon. With six weeks to go before the race, you'll need to put in the miles for a couple of Tuesday workouts. The long run is 18 miles, which you have done three times before so the distance isn't the issue, but rather the fact that you're going to try to run 6 of these miles at marathon pace, which I will discuss in a moment.

This is also the first time in the training where you are running assigned paces. Not only are you running marathon pace, but you will be running half marathon pace at times as well. Grooving your marathon pace is key, but having to "change gears" in the middle of marathon pace work and run half marathon pace is also an important part of the SMT system in the final weeks of marathon preparation.

So, how do you figure out what pace to run when marathon pace is assigned? Use the table in chapter seventeen to find your marathon pace.

The next thing you need to do is to use an online calculator, (go to *Resources* in the Appendix for a list of calculators) and see the corresponding half marathon pace. You will see that a general rule of thumb is that if you take the half marathon time, double it and add 10 minutes, this should correspond to the marathon time you're using. There are always runners who can run a great half marathon and can't run the corresponding marathon time that the rule of thumb predicts. The problem that these runners have is a lack of quality long runs and too little overall volume. This is not a problem you will have if you follow the SMT system.

You need to have both your MP and half marathon pace (HMP) calculated to execute Tuesday's workout. This is also the first Tuesday work where you will be using miles rather than minutes for the workout assignment. If your goal pace is 4 hours for the marathon, this workout is going to take you quite a bit longer than workouts up to this point. Make sure you have enough time in your day to get in both the workout and the SAM Hard work without being rushed.

Tuesday's workout is 2 miles easy, then 4 miles at marathon pace. This should feel good, as you're only running 4 miles at a pace you will be able to run for 26.2 miles. After the 4 miles at MP section, you will switch gears and run 1 mile at HMP. This does two things. First, it raises the intensity of the workout, helping you get a greater aerobic stimulus. Second, it gets you out of the groove of marathon pace, specifically your unique biomechanics at marathon pace. Now you might be thinking, "You said that the reason to run MP was to groove the pace." Yes, that's true, but with six weeks to go in training, you can get into a rut with running MP if that's all you do. You want MP to feel good, or at least feel doable in the workouts where you are fatigued and running MP. The very subtle difference in biomechanics, e.g. knee lift and arm angles, make this a great workout at this point in the 20-week training cycle. After the 1 mile at HMP, you go back to 3 miles at MP. The objective is to get back into the groove of MP. Finish the workout with 1 mile easy.

The first couple of minutes running MP following the HMP you may be a bit fatigued, but you will feel better and better throughout the second 3 mile section, as the pace is slower. This is an opportunity to practice running relaxed when you are running MP. What you're trying to do is groove the rhythm of MP. Rhythm is so important for a runner, as is learning to run a specific pace/rhythm when you are uncomfortable. That's what this workout teaches you to do. Finish with 1 mile easy, then right into SAM Hard.

Key Point

Do not think about having to run MP for 26.2 miles in these marathon workouts. It is so easy to get intimidated by MP when you're only doing it for a handful of miles. The workout this week is much more challenging than it looks. Couple this with the fact that you are not rested, but rather in the midst of difficult marathon training, you're likely not going to feel comfortable running MP at this point in the training. Trust the SMT system! It works, and come race day you'll be muscularly strong, aerobically fit, and your legs will feel fresh. The reality is that you are six weeks away from race day and now is the time to train. You're training on tired legs now, but when you begin to taper (starting in Week Eighteen), your legs will soon feel fresh and snappy, and MP will feel completely different, especially in the first 10, 15, and 20 miles of the marathon.

Wednesday is another 60-90 minute run. This is the last Wednesday where you will have this long of an assignment. As long as you get in 60 minutes easy you've had a great *tired legs run*, yet if you're feeling like you want a bonus and can go 90, you've got the green light. This makes for a wonderful two-day training block of Tuesday/Wednesday. Money in the bank.

Saturday is going to be a challenge—an 18-mile run—which you know by now is a challenging distance. The good news is that there's nothing to be intimidated by. At this point in the training you've run an 18-mile run three times, and you've run beyond 18 miles twice.

This week the goal is to execute an 18-mile run with MP running in the middle of it. 11 miles easy, 6 miles at marathon pace, finishing with 1 mile easy. A straightforward assignment, but not an easy one. If you get to the 11-mile mark and don't feel well then just get in the 18-mile run. That's a good day and you won't be behind in your training by running an 18-mile run rather than 18 miles with some MP running in the middle. That said, most athletes I've worked with are able to do the MP running, even in the midst of the training volume, which is high at this point. Again, don't think about the fact that you will be running MP for 26.2 miles. Running 6 miles at MP from mile 11 to mile 17 is a great stimulus. While it will be a mental challenge to knock out the SAM Hard routines after this run, it's vital that you do so this week. I know, I know, everything is vital and necessary. Trust the system; the interlinking aspects of training is the special sauce of the SMT system. Eighteen miles with 6 miles at MP, followed by SAM Hard is the most challenging day to date in your training. Celebrate with a glass of water at the end of your workout!

Oh yeah, I almost forgot. A brisk walk on Sunday please. If something comes up in your life and you can only fit in 30 minutes, that's fine, *but you cannot skip the walk* as your legs will not be ready for the challenges of Week Sixteen if you do.

Week 16

This week is simple. You need to run 22 miles on Saturday. You need to do this for the simple reason that your body has the ability, if you give it the proper stimulus, to burn fat, a vital fuel source during the marathon. The 22-mile run gives your body a great stimulus to facilitate this process. Runners who run a strong 22-mile run in their training run solid marathons on race day. Period. So this is exactly what you're going to do. I said it was simple—now for the details of all the simplicity.

To run a strong 22-mile run, you need to be rested going into the run. With this in mind, you will have five days, Monday through Friday, that will all be a bit easier than your normal week. Monday you will only run 50 minutes. Tuesday the total workout is 80 minutes, but it's a very easy workout. Wednesday you will only run 60 minutes. Thursday is 10 minutes less cross training than normal. Friday is just 40 minutes, compared to the normal 50 minute run. The cumulative effect of this rest is that you will be ready to not only run 22 miles on Saturday, but you will be able to run strong for the entire distance.

M   LMLS, 50 minutes easy with 5 x 30 second strides (60-90 seconds easy recovery), SAM Easy.

T   LMLS, 10-minute warm-up, 40 minutes at MP, then 5 minutes "fun-fast," finishing with 15 minutes at MP, 10-minute cool-down, then SAM Hard.

W   LMLS, 60 minutes easy, SAM Easy.

Th LMLS, 35-50 minutes easy cross training, SAM Easy.

F   LMLS, 40 minutes easy with 5 x 30 second strides (60-90 seconds easy recovery), SAM Easy.

S   LMLS, 22 miles easy, the longest run of the training cycle, making sure to run the first 10 miles conservatively, then SAM Easy (not SAM Hard).

Su Brisk walk of 60-90 minutes, LMLS before and SAM Easy afterward is encouraged. Also, 20-30 minutes of easy walking in the evening is encouraged.

WEEK 16

Tuesday will be a very light day. The workout is simply 40 minutes at marathon pace, no problem, then 5 minutes when you get to run *fun fast*. I can hear you saying it, "Oh, goody two shoes! *Fun fast*, hooray!" Let me explain all the fun. *Fun fast* is a pace that is faster than half marathon pace. Just run faster than HMP for 5 minutes and you've got yourself *fun fast*. That's it. Feel good, have fun, and go back to the groove of MP for another 15 minutes. MP will feel very comfortable after 5 minutes of *fun fast* running. While this workout is a total of 80 minutes, it's not a challenging workout. You follow this workout with 60 minutes on Wednesday, making the two days both less intense and shorter in volume than your recent Tuesday/Wednesday workout combinations. Thursday and Friday are very easy. A 40-minute run on Friday will go by quickly. Spend some of this run getting mentally ready for the task of the 22-mile run.

So how do you run 22 miles? The first thing you need to do is to prepare for the run by selecting a course that is less than 22 miles. As I've mentioned before, you want to have the ability to cut the run to 18 or 20 miles if you're having a bad day for whatever reason. Long runs get exponentially harder as the length increases. A 22-mile run is much more difficult than a 20-mile run. We don't want you to dig a hole for yourself because of one tough run, resulting in several days trying to get your energetic self back. Yes, the 22-mile run will be intense and require several recovery days, but the concern here is that if you feel poor at the 18-mile mark, and feel horrible at 20 miles, then it makes sense for you to stop. Better to get in a 20-mile day where you dig only a shallow hole for yourself, than get in 22 miles where you dig a deep hole for yourself, requiring a week or longer to recover.

GEEK OUT
Read more about The Science of Optimizing Fueling During the Marathon on page 197

The good news is, the vast majority of athletes not only run the 22-mile run, but they are able to run it strong due to the training up to this point. At this point in your training, 22 miles is a realistic Saturday run and you simply need to mentally focus and prepare for the logistics.

Not only do you need to plan out the course you're going to run, you need to plan out your fueling. When are your going to take gels and sports drinks on race day? Set up cups of water on tables or your car hood somewhere along the course. Today you must practice your fueling strategy for race day. If you need some guidance in this area make sure to read Dr. Trent Stellingwerff's Geek Out on the Science of Optimizing Fueling During the Marathon on page 197. Please note, there is an approach to doing long runs where you purposely don't take gels or sports drink, called *the glycogen-depleted long run*. This type of run isn't part of the SMT system for this particular marathon schedule, but can be considered in some of the advanced schedules.

Once you have your course laid out and a plan for your fueling, then you're ready to execute the run. The key is to start conservatively. You can always speed up at the end of the run. You will have a horrible experience if you go out too hard in the first 10-15 miles of the run and then painfully shuffle your way through the final miles. This is one of the few days where it will make sense to check your watch each mile for the first few miles. Ten to fifteen seconds a mile slower than your normal long run pace is a good rule of thumb for the first 10 miles of the run. Once you get 10 miles under your belt, there is a good chance you will feel like running normal long run pace for the remainder of the run.

This run should give you the confidence that you can run longer than 20 miles and feel strong both mentally and physically. Resist the urge to speculate about pace, things like, "How am I going to run MP, which is a much faster pace than I ran today, on race day?" *Do not* let your mind ask these questions. This is very important. This run should give you confidence that you can run a strong marathon. The run should not cause doubt or anxiety about your ability to run the distance. If you trust the training, you'll get to race day ready to execute your best 26.2-mile race. Find solace in the fact that you still have a month of training during which you will simultaneously continue to gain fitness and start the process of resting for the race.

The goal of this run is simple: finish 22 miles. Pace does not matter. In fact, there are some schools of thought that recommend you should do one run during your marathon preparation that is the same duration as the time you will run in the marathon. While we won't make this a particular goal, it's worth noting that the 22-mile run will, for most runners, get them close to their projected finish time for the marathon.

If you run conservatively for the first 18 miles and find yourself feeling good at the 18-mile mark, there is no reason to speed up. Just stay on pace and run strong through the remaining 4 miles. The ideal way to end this run is to finish strong enough to say, "I'm so glad to be done with the run, but I know I could have run 1-2 more miles at that pace if I had to." Most runners I've worked with have had this experience on the 22-mile run for the simple fact that they've done the training up to this point and they are therefore prepared for a great run.

This is the one long run that you can do SAM Easy after. You need to get in the SAM but you don't need to have a killer session. Getting the SAM Easy work immediately after the run has a tremendous benefit, but make sure you take a minute or two and take in some fluids in the form of water or a recovery drink to get through the last few minutes of the SAM work. This is particularly important after the 22-mile run.

You will need to plan most of your Saturday around this run. The run takes up all of the morning, then you need to get in some quality calories, and finally, you will probably want a nap. A great way to nap is to be in your bed, with the lights out, door closed, shades drawn, and an alarm, just as you would if you were going to sleep. At least, that's how I like it. If you prefer and can do it, fall asleep on the couch in front of a TV. However you need to, take a nap. Trust me, you won't need much more than getting yourself horizontal for a few minutes and you'll be out.

You will be walking briskly on Sunday, the normal 60-90 minute assignment. You should also consider going for a gentle walk Saturday evening after the 22-mile run, if only for 20 or 30 minutes. A walk in the evening after the 22-mile run helps most runners' legs feel better. If you have the time, I highly suggest the Saturday evening gentle walk in addition to your Sunday morning brisk walk.

TRAINING WEEKS 17-20:

GROOVE MARATHON PACE
——— TO HAVE A GREAT RACE ———

"Of course motivation is not
permanent. But then neither is
bathing, but it is something you
should do on a regular basis."

— Zig Zigler

CHAPTER 10

Week 17

The importance of this week in the 20-week training cycle is that you spend the first two days of the week recovering from the 22-mile run. Thank you for trusting the importance of this run in the SMT system, and thank you for trusting that you need intentional rest following the intensity that this long run presents.

Your ability to run well on race day is directly related to the 22-mile run. The first few days of Week Seventeen are designed to help you recover from the intense run and have you ready to train injury-free. You must recover from the 22-mile run if you're going to be able to train well for the last four weeks. It's an easy week until you get to Saturday, where you need to run 16 miles with 8 miles at marathon pace. The 16-mile run is arguably as important as the 22-mile run, as you run 8 miles at MP in the second half of the run, then immediately into SAM Hard following the run.

M   Complete day off from running and cross training.

T   LMLS, 45 minutes easy with 5 x 30 second strides (60-90 seconds easy recovery), SAM Easy.

W   LMLS, 60-70 minutes easy, SAM Easy.

Th   LMLS, 45-60 minutes easy cross training, SAM Easy.

F   LMLS, 50 minutes easy with 5 x 30 second strides (60-90 seconds easy recovery), SAM Easy.

S   LMLS, 16 mile long run: 7 miles easy, 8 miles at MP, 1 mile cool-down, then immediately into SAM Hard.

Su   Brisk walk of 60-90 minutes, LMLS before and SAM Easy afterward is encouraged.

WEEK 17

Monday is one of the few days of complete rest in the SMT system. You need to take this day completely off. No running, no cross training, no brisk walk, and no SAM work. You can do leg swings and mobility work from SAM Easy, but none of the general strength work (e.g., planks). Ideally, this is a day you would see an Active Release Techniques (A.R.T.) professional. A.R.T. therapists are, in my opinion, best equipped to help healthy runners stay healthy after running 22 miles two days prior. An A.R.T. therapist might be a physical therapist, a chiropractor, a massage therapist, or some other health care professional. The key is to find an A.R.T. therapist that works with endurance athletes and understands that you have to be able to run again this week. This is different than a massage therapist who may want to do deep tissue work. This kind of work has its place for runners, but 48 hours after a 22-mile run is not the time for invasive deep tissue work. You can find a list of A.R.T. professionals at *www.activerelease.com*.

Tuesday is not a workout, but rather a shorter version of a normal Monday: 45 minutes easy with strides. You need to use this day to take an inventory of your body,

GEEK OUT
Read more about Finding A Practitioner on page 192

making sure you don't have any acute pains, and making sure you aren't inappropriately sore. Some runners feel flat on this day until they get to the strides, which usually feel decent. Conversely, some runners feel great after 48 hours of very light activity. Regardless, you'll likely feel better on the Wednesday run. SAM Easy is the assignment for today, rather than SAM Hard. The bottom line is, while all of the Tuesdays leading up to this point have been workouts, we want today to be an easy recovery day.

Wednesday is simply 60-70 minutes and SAM Easy. You should be feeling close to 100% by today. 60 to seventy minutes is a solid run, but you've run 70 minutes or longer so many times by this point that it shouldn't be a tough day mentally. Thursday and Friday are back to normal volumes.

Saturday is an interesting run and one that you should be focused for, even though you will only run 16 miles. You will run 7 miles easy, then 8 miles at MP, then a 1 mile cool down. You need to do this on a flat course. If you've been doing your long runs on a hilly course, this means finding a shorter loop that is relatively flat and running the loop several times.

Your marathon will likely be on a flat course, and today you want to simulate running on the same topography as in the race. The 7 miles easy is self-explanatory. You can use mile 8 to gradually speed up until you hit MP. Continue MP pace until the 15-mile mark. The 8 miles of MP will be tough, no doubt, but you can do it.

This workout is one of the best stimuli you'll get during the 20 weeks of SMT training, but just like the 22-mile run, you must not think about the fact that you will be running MP for 26.2 miles. Get the 8 miles at MP done and don't worry about how you feel. If you feel great, fantastic! If you feel horrible, that's fine, don't worry about it. You don't need to feel great to reap the benefits of this run, you just need to get the stimulus. In my experience, roughly 25% of people feel so-so on this run and 75% of people feel strong, which is interesting when you consider that virtually everyone who follows the SMT system runs well on race day.

Feeling good on this run is not a predictor of success on race day; merely finishing this run is a predictor of success on marathon day. SAM Hard immediately after the run makes this the most challenging SAM Hard assignment you will do over the course of the 20-week training cycle. Be focused, be energetic, and simply knock it out. What a day! A long run, a significant amount of MP running, and a very challenging SAM Hard stimulus makes for a big day. You're now well on your way to having the fitness and toughened mindset necessary for a solid marathon performance. Sunday's brisk walk is, as always, important given the intensity of Saturday.

Week 18

In Week Eighteen you start the process of resting for the race, which is called the taper. The term taper is a bit broad and means different things to different coaches.

I want you to think of two variables when you think of the taper: volume and intensity. We are going to slowly decrease the volume you're running from now until race day, but we aren't going to decrease the intensity quite as much. I'll jump ahead to this week's long run to give you an example. The run is 14 miles, shorter than what you've been doing. The run has 7 miles at MP in the middle of it, making this 14-mile run challenging. Saturday is shorter than usual, but still a challenging assignment based on the intensity of the MP running.

The other two key elements of the taper that are important are: MP running; and rest and recovery, not only after the hard days, but every day. While no one will expect that your life will be completely stress-free over the next three weeks, aim for a bedtime 10-20 minutes earlier than normal. After two or three weeks of going to bed earlier you will begin to feel the benefit. Good recovery means good hydration and good fueling, so you need to make sure you're eating well and hydrating properly between workouts. MP running in these final three weeks comes down to a simple reality: You are fit and you have put in the long runs for a good marathon. The only missing piece is to spend even more time at marathon pace, making it as comfortable as possible.

M	LMLS, 55 minutes with 5 x 30 second strides (60-90 seconds easy recovery), SAM Easy.
T	LMLS, 2 miles warm-up, 4 miles at MP, 1 mile at HMP, 3 miles at MP, 1 mile cool-down, SAM Hard.
W	LMLS, 60-70 minutes easy, SAM Easy.
Th	LMLS, 45-60 minutes easy cross training, SAM Easy.
F	LMLS, 45-50 minutes easy with 5 x 30 second strides (60-90 seconds easy recovery), SAM Easy.
S	LMLS, 14 mile long run: 6 miles easy, 7 miles at MP, 1 mile cool-down, SAM Hard immediately after the run.
Su	Brisk walk of 60 minutes, LMLS before and SAM Easy afterward is encouraged.

Monday is a normal training day of 55 minutes. Next week will be 50 minutes, but this week you should stay at 55. Tuesday is a marathon pace workout, with some half marathon pace running in the middle. Specifically, you'll run 4 miles at MP, then 1 mile at HMP, finishing with 3 miles at MP. Just as you did in Weeks Fifteen and Sixteen, you're running MP, then speeding up for a bit, then going to back to MP to groove the pace.

Why are you doing this workout? Simple: the projected marathon pace (MP) needs to be deeply *grooved* into your being. You need your entire body to be comfortable with the specific biomechanics of running your MP, from your big toe to the top of your head! You need to learn to be as relaxed as possible running this pace. You're fit enough to run this pace for a marathon, but getting your mind ready to stay relaxed at this pace in the early miles is the first task. In the final 6.2 miles of the race it will be up to you to be mentally tough in order to sustain this pace as you become more and more uncomfortable.

It's very easy to fall into negative self-talk in this workout as you begin to wonder if you can run MP for 26.2 miles, or, if you're really faltering, begin to wonder why you're doing this at all. Turn your mind off and just get in the MP running without worrying about how you feel. Most athletes feel very good in this workout, but in the rare case that you do not, keep the faith that come race day you can run MP for the entire 26.2-mile distance.

Regardless of how you feel on the run, you will be able to recover the next day. Remember, we are keeping the intensity high at this point in the training cycle, so both men and women should do SAM Hard. We will give a small tweak to the SAM days, according to gender, in Weeks Nineteen and Twenty. You might be surprised to learn that women get less of a break on SAM work than men do. Of course this isn't because the SMT system prefers men and wants to lavish special treatment. The difference has to do with women's physiology that tends to have a different response to the taper.

Wednesdays are crucial both this week and in Week Nineteen. *When in doubt, do less* (#WIDDL). Wednesdays have been important up to this point, but in these last two weeks they aren't nearly as important as you begin to feel energetic, with fresh legs. Week Eighteen Wednesday is 60-70 minutes easy. There is definitely no need to run longer than 70 minutes. If for some reason you don't feel well at the 60-minute mark, please stop the run and call it a day.

Thursday is 45-60 minutes of cross training. If in doubt, do 45 minutes. Friday is 45-50 minutes, and again, if in doubt do 45 minutes.

Saturday is a run that you can execute and feel good about: 14 miles, with the first 6 miles easy, then gradually speeding up to MP for 7 miles. Finish with a 1-mile cool-down. SAM Hard for both genders this week, though next Saturday (Week Nineteen) this will change.

This workout has the same positives and negatives as Tuesday. You need this run, both for its volume and intensity. But you also need this run mentally. Most runners feel strong after this run, and even though you won't run 14 miles at MP, the fact that you get to mile 13 of a run and you're running MP and feeling good is a definite confidence builder.

This week the brisk walk is only 60 minutes. Catch up on some extra sleep, but don't look at the shortened walk as time to spend a couple hours doing yard work or spend an afternoon on your feet shopping. You are tapering and you need to be resting. Save these domestic activities until after the marathon.

Week 19

This is the last week that will look like normal training. The volume is decreased each day, but the structure of the week stays the same. Tuesday is a straight forward workout and Saturday is similar to last week, but you will run less, only 12 miles, with 6 of these miles at MP.

Again, if you can get just 10-20 minutes more rest each night, it will positively impact your training. This is the week where you can start the imagery process for race day, as seeing the race well in advance is a key component to running a great race.

Note: SAM Easy for men on Saturday; SAM Hard for women on Saturday.

M   LMLS, 50 minutes easy with 5 x 30 second strides (60-90 seconds easy recovery), SAM Easy.

T   LMLS, 2 miles warm-up, 3 miles at MP, 0.5 miles "fun-fast," 3 miles at MP, 1 mile cool-down, SAM Hard.

W   LMLS, 60 minutes easy, SAM Easy.

Th   LMLS, 45 minutes easy cross training, SAM Easy.

F   LMLS, 45 minutes easy with 5 x 30 second strides (60-90 seconds easy recovery), SAM Easy.

S   LMLS, 12 mile long run: 5 miles easy, 6 miles at MP, 1 mile cool-down, SAM immediately after the run (SAM Easy for men, SAM Hard for women).

Su   Brisk walk of 45 minutes, LMLS before and SAM Easy afterward is encouraged.

WEEK 19

Monday is just 50 minutes this week. Trust the subtle drop in volume. Tuesday is a simple workout, 10 miles total. A 2-mile warm-up, 3 miles at MP, a half mile at *fun fast* pace, 3 miles at MP, and a 1 mile cool-down.

The goal of this workout is twofold. First, you need a bit of running before the marathon that is faster than race pace. While you get this in the form of strides on your easy days, running the *fun fast* half mile is a great way to challenge your neuromuscular system and get you into slightly different biomechanics than your marathon pace. The second goal of this workout is that in the 3 MP miles following the *fun fast* half mile, you need to settle down and run MP. In the first couple of minutes of MP you're going to be tired; this is to be expected. By the end of the 3 miles at MP you'll be feeling good. This run is a great stimulus this close to the race: grooving marathon pace, changing to a slightly challenging pace, and then settling back down to MP and grooving again. Athletes love this workout because it's short, it's fun, and the 3 miles at MP to end the workout feel very comfortable.

The only potential problem here is that you have to make sure that *fun fast* doesn't accidentally become *hard fast*. It should be fun, and should be a pace you can run for 2 or 3 miles and have just as much fun. SAM on this day is normal for women. If you're a male and your legs have been sore the past few weeks, then take out the challenging lower body work and do the rest of the SAM routine.

GEEK OUT
Read more about Using Imagery To Run Your Best marathon on page 187

Wednesday is a 60-minute run. There is no need to do more than 60 minutes. Remember, we are tapering and half of this equation means that you are running fewer minutes in the week than you did earlier in the training. For most athletes, this is an enjoyable run as the legs are starting to feel good.

This week, cross train for 45 minutes on Thursday and run 45 minutes on Friday. Don't accidentally bump up the effort on these days. You'll likely feel great on Friday, so keep the pace in check, running your normal easy day pace.

Saturday is your last long run, and it's not very long at 12 miles. The goal of the run is exactly the same as Tuesday, just a couple of miles longer. Five miles easy, 6 miles at marathon pace, and a 1-mile cool-down. This is basically the same run as last Saturday in

GEEK OUT
Read more about Practice Makes Perfect (or at least better prepared) on page 194

terms of how you approach it. You need to get in some MP work and you need to do it within the context of a longer run, but overall this is not a difficult run, as you're fit and ready to race. As I've said for all of the MP running, don't spend time wondering if you can run MP for 26.2 miles. You can, even if you don't feel great on this particular training run. Most athletes feel great, with their overall energy high and their legs feeling rested.

At this point in the training schedule the SAM assignments diverge based on gender. Men should do SAM Easy today, while women should do SAM Hard. We want a final SAM Hard stimulus for women to keep a hormonal profile of high testosterone and high human growth hormone going into the race. While body builders have these hormones in greater quantities than runners, the SAM work will keep these hormone levels higher compared to runners who have done no general strength. I learned this concept as a collegiate coach. I lowered the amount of SAM in the taper for both collegiate and professional athletes and the result was that the female athletes felt flat at the competition.

If you're a woman reading this, you need to knock out this last SAM Hard session and trust that it's going to help you on race day. Men have higher levels of testosterone and human growth hormone, so doing SAM Easy is one more day to rest the legs before the race. But women shouldn't worry about their legs being heavy on race day from this one stimulus. Your legs no doubt feel rested at this point in the training and they are going to feel even better next week.

Obviously you need a brisk walk on Sunday to deal with the stress of Saturday, but you only need to go for 45 minutes.

Week 20

You've arrived at race week! After a simple workout on Tuesday, the rest of the week is in service of keeping your legs fresh and poppy, and to remind your body that when the gun goes off, you'll *groove and grind* a great race. No reason to make this week complicated. This is the easiest week of training in the entire 20-week training cycle. Stay on top of your sleep and find time each day during this week for a short imagery session. Both are going to help you when the gun goes off.

The major goal for this week is singular: to race well on Sunday. To do this, you need to focus on getting a proper amount of rest throughout the week, trusting that the training you've done up to this point is enough.

Every running day of this week will be shorter than what you've done in the past, with the added bonus of the day off on Thursday, 72 hours before the race.

M   LMLS, 40 minutes easy with 5 x 30 second strides (60-90 seconds easy recovery), SAM Easy.

T   LMLS, 1 mile warm-up, 2 miles at MP, 1 mile at HMP, 3 miles at MP, 1 mile cool-down, SAM Easy.

W   LMLS, 35-40 minutes easy with 5 x 30 second strides (60-90 seconds easy recovery), SAM Easy.

Th   Complete day off from running and cross training.

F   LMLS, 30-35 minutes easy, SAM Easy.

S   Pre-race, 10-15 minute easy running, then 5 x 30 second strides (60-90 seconds easy recovery), then 5-minute cool-down, LS and hip mobility from Phase 1 SAM Easy.

Su   Race! Execute a smart race plan and you'll be happy with the result. Remember, be conservative in the opening miles of the race.

WEEK 20

Monday is 40 minutes easy and strides. You are rested and your legs are feeling good at this point, so you must make sure not to accidentally run faster than normal. Do the entire SAM Easy routine today, and every day, up to race day.

Tuesday is not a hard workout. At first glance it might look like it's long, but it's not. It's 8 miles total, a distance you will recover from the next day. One mile warm-up, 2 miles at MP, then 1 mile at half marathon pace (HMP), 3 miles at MP, 1-mile cool-down. You know the rationale: we want MP to feel comfortable after having run HMP. The goal is to feel as comfortable as possible running the two MP portions, especially the second portion. This is a great last workout because it's long enough to remind your body that Sunday is a big challenge, yet it's short enough that you'll be recovered the next day. SAM Easy at the end of the run.

Wednesday is a replica of Monday, but 35 minutes rather than 40 minutes. Doing some strides is a great way to get the legs moving fast, with the effect that MP will feel like an easy-going pace.

Thursday is a day off. Even though it might not feel intuitive to take the day off, you need to. Trust me and trust this important day in the SMT system. If you're feeling anxious and you must do something, you can do the mobility work from SAM. That's it. At this point in the training schedule, the work is done. Don't even think about cramming. Cramming might work for some people on exams, but it does not work for anyone running a marathon.

Friday calls for a 30 to 35-minute run and SAM Easy. Enjoy this run. This is a day where you also need to be careful not to run too fast. Just a nice, easy run, enjoying the energetic, snappy leg feeling you have now that you are completely rested. You should feel a bit of pent up energy, as if you'd really like to be let off the leash. Don't let yourself off the leash until Sunday.

Saturday is pre-race day. You will do 10 to 15 minutes of warm-up running, then your normal 5 x 30 second strides, and 5 minutes of cool-down running. Finish with leg swings and the mobility exercises from SAM (no general strength, such as planks). You need to find a safe place to do the strides (sometimes this is hard if you're racing in a city). Scout this out before your run.

Spend as little time in the expo area as possible. Many runners compromise months of training by spending hours shopping for gear and checking out the latest running gadgets. Resist this urge! You can shop some other time. If you need to go to the expo to pick up your packet, get in and out as quickly as possible. If you need to buy some gear to commemorate the race, fine, but don't get sucked into the expo. You've been tapering to get your legs feeling fresh and ready to race. Don't undo this crucial aspect of the taper by spending too much time on your feet at the expo.

Sunday is the day you've been working towards for twenty weeks. The key to Sunday is to be as calm and collected as possible in the hours before the race. You will likely be a little nervous, and you should be; this is a race, not a long run. However, you'll need to manage your nerves. Nervousness that becomes anxiety will hurt your performance. Belly breathing and using imagery as relaxation tools will help calm your nerves. No need to worry at this point, you've done all the difficult workouts and long runs. The money is in the bank. You're prepared for this race. Recall all the long runs you've done. All the SAM you've sweated through. All the MP running you've done.

Take it easy on race day, stay off your feet. When it's the appropriate time, you'll begin the warm-up. You'll need just 3-5 minutes of jogging and a few strides, basically the least amount of running necessary to increase your body temperature and get in some 5k pace strides so the MP feels comfortable.

The next chapter is devoted entirely to race day and I'll go into detail regarding your plan for the race and how to execute a great race. You've put in twenty weeks of great training and now it's time to race!

—— RACE DAY ——

"Perfection is not attainable.
But if we chase perfection, we
can catch excellence."

— Vince Lombardi

CHAPTER 11

I f you've followed the SMT system and put in all of the work, you are now capable of running a marathon to your potential. This is exciting! That said, you still have to execute a sound race plan if you're going to race to your potential. I am confident that the skills you've learned in the twenty weeks leading up to the race, namely the skill of running by feel, will help you execute the race plan I'm about to lay out.

You've taught your body how to utilize fat as a fuel source, an attribute that's going to keep you from "hitting the wall" around mile 20 (no small thing), allowing you to run strong in the final miles of the race. If you've had muscle cramping issues in previous marathons, there is a very good chance that these days are behind you as the SAM work, which you've been so diligently doing, has made your legs exceedingly strong and ready to handle the 26.2 miles of pounding without withering. The bottom line is, you're fit and healthy, and it's time to race smart and run fast.

Groove And Grind: A Simple Plan For Race Day

Recall with me the meaning of *groove and grind* mentioned a few chapters back. You want to *groove* marathon pace for 20 miles and then *grind* out the last 6.2 miles. You've run so many long runs that running strong for the first 20 miles will not be a problem. However, you must make sure that in the opening miles of the race you do not accidentally run 5-10 seconds a mile faster than your MP. If you were to run 10 seconds a mile too fast in the first 18 miles of the race, it would put you 3 minutes ahead of your goal time.

This might sound like a smart plan: get a little bit ahead so that if the final 6.2 miles are tough, you will still hit your goal. *This is absolutely the wrong thing to do.* Rather, you must be disciplined and run as close to MP as possible in the opening miles, which will allow you to maintain MP for the final 6.2 miles of the race (and you may even speed up in these final miles). Coming through the 18 mile mark three minutes ahead of your MP almost always means you will struggle to maintain MP in the final 6.2 miles. I've had clients go out too fast in the first 18 miles of the race, running as much as a minute per mile slower in the final miles, meaning that they could end up running 3-8 minutes slower than their goal finishing time. Don't let this be your story on race day.

How do you keep things under control and run MP in the first 20 miles of the race? If you have a GPS watch that will beep when exceeding MP, this would be ideal. Or, you can check your splits at each mile mark. By mile 5 of the race you should be settled into your MP rhythm, ready to focus on the race ahead of you.

Now that we have established that you aren't going to compromise your race by going out too fast, let's talk about grooving the pace for the first 20 miles. It's just as it sounds. Your body, through proper training, is ready to run MP for 20 miles and feel strong doing it. That said, be ready for the random mile or two in the first 20 when you'll have to stay mentally focused to stay on pace. As my friend Zach Hancock, a former 4:03 collegiate miler and 2:57 marathoner, has said about the marathon and long-distance nordic ski races, "There are lots of races in the race." This will be true in the first 20 miles of the race. You'll likely hit a tough mile and will need to focus in order to "win" this race within the race.

When you get to mile 20 there is a very good chance that you'll feel strong. Even if you've felt strong up to this point, this is the place in the race where you'll have to start to *grind*. The reality is, the marathon, when raced well, is a grueling task. You're not going to race to your potential and feel great the entire way. Once you start to feel uncomfortable, you simply need to focus.

GEEK OUT
Read more about You Do Hard Things on page 182

I encourage you to use the language that my friend Cindy Kuzma uses, which is, "You do hard things." Self-talk is powerful. When you speak this phrase to yourself, you accept the hard task and prepare yourself to grind out the pace to the finish line.

While there are many ways to approach the last 6.2 miles of the race, a simple way to "chunk" the task is as follows: when you hit 20 miles, you say, "I'm going to focus on the next 3 miles and I'm going to grind." When you've completed these 3 miles and you're at the 23 mile mark you say, "I'm going to try to speed up by a quarter of a notch and grind out the next 2 miles." Why try to speed up? Because if you don't mentally ask your body to speed up at this juncture, there is a very good chance that you will slow just a bit. Tell yourself to speed up to stay on pace.

GEEK OUT
Read more about The Last 6.2 miles of a Marathon on page 195

When you hit the 25-mile mark, the final task left is to grind out the last 1.2 miles of the race, arriving at the finish as fast as you can. Yes, you're going to be uncomfortable, but you're fit and your muscularly strong – you can do this! And it's fun, in a marathon sort of way.

So, this is the simple plan. Be cautious not to accidentally run faster than MP in the opening miles. Groove your marathon pace for 20 miles, and then grind out the last 6.2 miles, breaking it up into three mental segments: 3 miles, 2 miles, and a 1.2-mile segment. That's it! Do these things and you'll run a great race that will make you grateful for all of the hard work you have put in.

GEEK OUT
Read more about The Sciences of Fueling, Heat Acclimation, and Hydration on pages 197-208

There are three technical Geek Out sections that you'll want to read at some point, all written by one of the best physiologists in the world, Dr. Trent Stellingwerff. These sections ensure you have a plan for fueling and hydration, as well as a plan in case you find yourself running in warm and/or humid conditions.

RECOVERY CYCLE:

FOUR WEEKS —— THAT COULD —— CHANGE YOUR RUNNING

"Nature does not hurry,
yet everything is accomplished."

— Lao Tzu

CHAPTER 12

This is a very straightforward chapter, with a very simple message. The recovery cycle after a marathon is an opportunity to become a better runner through the principle of *non-doing*—the Taoist principle of wu wei—action that does not involve struggle or excessive effort. You will do very little running in the four weeks following the marathon. The vast majority of people rush into training too soon after they finish a marathon, and this is a huge mistake. For some it's that they have trouble functioning in their daily lives without running, while others want to race, motivated by an erroneous belief that they need to get back to serious training to stay in shape and perpetuate previous training. I promise you that if you follow the four-week recovery cycle in this book, you will properly prepare yourself for the next block of serious training, be it training for a 5k, a marathon, or something else like a triathlon or an ultra marathon.

The SMT recovery cycle is a mix of cross training days, several full days off from running, SAM, and slow gentle runs. The progression builds from one or two runs in your first week of the recovery cycle to four runs in the fourth week. After the fourth week you can resume normal training in pursuit of whatever the next race goal might be.

The situation regarding recovery after a marathon is this: very few people want to take four easy weeks following the marathon, even though many of these people are aware of the popular concept that you need one day off from training for every mile that you raced. Standard wisdom advises a marathoner to take twenty-six days to recover. The recovery cycle that I am recommending is twenty-eight days of recovery with slow runs included.

The runner who is too impatient to properly recover from the marathon is often injured six to ten weeks after the marathon. The typical scenario goes something like this: initially the easier workouts and runs after the marathon are manageable, but soon the training gets more intense and the fragile post-marathon body, which has not been allowed to properly rejuvenate, begins to break down. This discouraging scenario doesn't have to be you if you follow a proper recovery cycle.

An added benefit to the recovery cycle is that it's a great time to start learning the AIF rope stretching, if you didn't already do so during the 20-week training cycle. Spending less time working out each day in the first couple weeks of the recovery cycle, you will create time to get in some rope stretching.

Habits take time to establish and the four-week recovery cycle is a great time to create a new habit; you can incorporate this new habit into your routine when you resume serious training.

Pool running is another unique aspect of the recovery cycle. The pool is a critical aspect of the cycle. When the pool is assigned you really need to take the time to find a pool. The recovery benefits of the hydrostatic pressure have been proven and will no doubt become more commonplace in the coming years.

Finally, you will be well served to see an A.R.T. professional once or twice a week during the recovery cycle. This type of work will set you up for injury-free training when you resume normal training. I think a good massage therapist, one who works with athletes, is an important piece of the puzzle for athletes who want to stay healthy over a training cycle and over years of running. That said, I advise that you avoid deep tissue massage in the first couple weeks of the recovery cycle. If you're someone who responds well to this type of therapy, then it can and should be utilized later in the recovery cycle.

GEEK OUT
Read more about Pool Walking on page 209

If you want to be running injury-free, and resume training at a high level after your marathon, it is vital that you take a short pause to properly recover. Four weeks of recovery is not a *nice to do, it's a need to do.*

WEEK 21

M	30-minute easy jog/walk to do a body scan and see what is sore and needs attention in the coming days.
T	Off, hip mobility from Phase 1 SAM Easy and AIF.
W	Brisk walk for 30-45 minutes.
Th	Cross train for 45 minutes, go very easy.
F	Off, hip mobility from Phase 2 SAM Easy and AIF.
S	LMLS, 35-minute easy run, SAM Easy.
Su	Brisk walk of 30-60 minutes.

WEEK 22

M	Cross train for 45 to 60 minutes easy.
T	LMLS, 30-minute easy run, SAM Easy, AIF.
W	Off, SAM Easy, AIF.
Th	Cross train for 45-60 minutes easy.
F	LMLS, 30-minute easy run, SAM Easy, AIF.
S	LMLS, 45-minute easy run, SAM Easy, AIF.
Su	Brisk walk of 45-60 minutes, SAM Easy, AIF.

WEEK 23

M	LMLS, 30-minute easy run, SAM Easy, AIF.
T	LMLS, 45-minute easy run, SAM Easy, AIF.
W	Off, SAM Easy and AIF.
Th	Cross train for 45 to 60 minutes easy.
F	LMLS, 35-minute easy run, SAM Easy, AIF.
S	LMLS, 60-minute easy run, SAM Easy, AIF.
Su	Brisk walk of 45-65 minutes, SAM Easy, AIF.

WEEK 24

M   LMLS, 45-minute run with 5 x 20 seconds at 5k pace with 90 seconds easy, SAM Easy.

T   LMLS, 60-minute easy run and if you feel good at 45 minutes, speed up for the last 15 minutes, then SAM "medium", which means you decide how much SAM to do.

W   LMLS, 45-minute easy run, SAM Easy.

Th Cross train easy for 45 to 60 minutes.

F   LMLS, 50 minutes with 5 x 20 seconds at 5k pace with 60 seconds easy, SAM Easy.

S   LMLS, 8 to 10 miles easy, just getting in the time on your feet, immediately into SAM Hard.

Su Brisk walk of 60-70 minutes.

WEEK 25

M   Back to normal training, LM, 45-50 minutes easy with 5 x 20 seconds at 5k pace with 60 seconds easy, SAM Easy.

THE
SELF-COACHED
RUNNER

— ● —   — ● —

"Run for fun and personal bests."

— Al Carius,
Men's Cross Country Coach
North Central College

CHAPTER 13

Make The Right Choices, Avoid Common Mistakes

There are many opportunities in the SMT system to make the right choice, leading to a better performance on race day. The flip side is you can unnecessarily push the training, ignore fatigue, and suffer from the stress factors (and potential stress fractures) that are impacting your training.

If you're a type-A personality, making the right choice (which 90% of the time means running slower or not running at all) will be difficult. If you truly want to improve as a runner, you will be willing to *do things you've never done before, so you can do things you've never done before* (such as running a PR).

If you've ever run a marathon and been less than satisfied with your performance, then not only is the SMT system going to help you have a great race, but you can help yourself within the system by paying attention to how you feel each and every day. With this in mind, let's look at some common examples of where you, the self-coached runner, can make the right choice.

Making The Right Choice On Wednesday

Simple problem: you run too hard on Tuesday and you don't end the workout saying, "I could have run one more repetition," or, "I could have run a little faster." You've run an effort that is closer to a race effort rather than a challenging, but controlled effort.

For illustrative purposes, let's say that the Wednesday assignment is as follows: LMLS, 75-minute run (if you feel good at the 45-minute mark, you can speed up a bit for the last 30 minutes), finish with SAM Easy.

What is the right choice in this scenario? Because you ran close to race effort on Tuesday, you start Wednesday with tired, heavy legs, and feeling tired in general. You get to the 45-minute mark and you don't feel better, yet you think to yourself, "I have 30 more minutes to run and I'm tired." The first mistake happens at this point. At the 45-minute mark you should make the right choice and say, "I'm not going to run 75 minutes today, I'm simply going to get in 60 minutes." Yet, so many runners go ahead and complete 75 minutes when they should simply get in 60 minutes, call it a day, and start the process of being ready to have a great long run on Saturday. At this point in the decision making process, the returns on work begin to diminish. The more times the wrong decision is made in succession, the faster the returns diminish.

In this scenario, running 75 minutes on Wednesday when you're fatigued is a bad idea and might well start a cycle of overtraining. Sure, you *should* be able to recover from Tuesday and Wednesday by the time you get to the Saturday long run, but there is also a chance that you'll start the long run fatigued and have a less than ideal run. I've said it throughout the book, but it's worth repeating: Make the right choice when you're tired, because the potential consequences of not doing so are too big to risk.

There is another lesson in the previous scenario. Please don't run so hard Tuesday that it becomes a race effort. Tuesday workouts aren't easy, but you should view them as challenging workouts that are controlled. Remember, you have a busy life, and when you do too much in training you don't have the luxury that professional athletes have of sleeping after a workout to be ready for the next challenging stimulus. A Tuesday when you choose to run too hard can be the start of a cascade of training where you are tired, lethargic, and prone to both sickness and injury.

The right choices are obvious. First, run hard but run controlled on Tuesday. If you fail to run controlled on Tuesday, then run easy on Wednesday and feel good about getting in 60 minutes. Sixty minutes is a solid but manageable run. Sixty minutes is always an option on Wednesday for the very reason that you need to do a solid effort but you need to avoid digging yourself a hole by running two days in a row that end up being hard days.

Remember, the SMT system is set up so that Tuesday is a significant challenge and Wednesday is a moderate challenge.

Make The Right Choice At All Times In The 20-Week Training Cycle!

The 20-week training cycle requires the self-coached running to make the right choice often, in many ways. The example I've highlighted throughout the book is making the right choice on Wednesday. It's the easiest example because if you feel fatigued after Tuesday's workout then you can simply run 60 minutes on Wednesday and feel good that you got in a solid run. We could come up with numerous examples where you need to make the right choice. For instance, you were up late finishing a project for work, or caring for a sick child, and when you wake up you're exhausted. Make the right choice and skip a day, even if it's Tuesday. If you wake up and you are sick, you need to take the day off to speed up the recovery process so that you can resume training. Just as you would need to be honest with a coach about what's happening in your life, you need to be honest with yourself.

Within workouts and long runs, there are going to be times when you need to make the right choice to both maximize the training effect of the SMT system and to prevent an overtraining cycle or undue stress to the body structurally (which could lead to an injury). For example, when you're doing Yasso 800s, don't run all-out on the last two 800s.

The assignment is to run 97% on the last one, not 100%. Even if the workout is going well and you want to see how fast you can run the final 800m repeat, make the right choice and finish strong, running hard, but not running all-out. If you're doing a long run and the assignment is to speed up the last 3 miles, don't run too hard in the last 3 miles. The assignment for these long runs is to speed up, but as with all of your runs, you need to be running controlled and you need to be able to say, "I definitely could have run 1 or 2 more miles." If you finish a long run and can't say this, you've made a mistake.

We could come up with many examples of making the right choice in training, but by now you get the point. The SMT system only works if you make the right choices at critical junctures throughout the training. Most of these junctures will be obvious, but some will be subtle. In both cases, you are capable of making the right choice, even if it's hard for you (e.g., the long run where you feel great and want to run fast at the end, yet you need to hold back a bit).

You can self-coach yourself well in the SMT system so long as you are in touch with the training and making the right choice at every juncture that calls for it. When you forget, re-read this chapter!

When In Doubt, Do Less (#WIDDL)

This one is simple. Regardless of the workout, *when in doubt, do less*. The best example of the *when in doubt, do less* concept is the weekly long run, when the assignment is to speed up in the last 3 miles. As you've read throughout chapters six through ten, the number one goal of the long run is to get in the distance assigned. That's it. Get in the run and feel good about your accomplishment when you finish the run. While you might be capable of speeding up at the end of every assigned run, there will be a few when you will doubt whether or not it is wise to do so. In these cases, do less and *don't speed up*. Live to fight another day.

If you've paid close attention in the last couple of chapters, you may recall that in the last three long runs before the race, you're assigned MP pace. You may be thinking, "How am I adhering to the SMT system training if I'm not running MP pace as part of my long runs when this is the assignment?" Fair question and here's the answer: if you get to the point in the run where you are supposed to speed up to MP and you're fatigued and can't imagine doing it, that's fine. Finish the run, do your SAM Hard work, get a shower and some good food, and enjoy the rest of your Saturday.

To be clear, by no means am I saying that over the course of a 20-week training cycle you should not speed up at the end of any of the runs. This would be a sign that you're training too hard on Tuesday and that your life stress is too high for you to be properly prepared for the crucial Saturday long run. However, on the one or two occasions that you have a long run and you are really fatigued, this is an opportunity to follow the *when in doubt, do less* principle.

Another example of *when in doubt, do less* is to simply not work out on Thursday if you're really fatigued from Tuesday and Wednesday. The SMT system is set up so that once, twice, perhaps three or four times in the 20-week training cycle, you simply take off Thursday. You will not lose fitness! When you get to Thursday and you're dragging, the key is to be honest about your energy level. By taking off Thursday, you give yourself the opportunity to feel good on Saturday, ready to run a solid long run. Taking a day off when there is an assigned workout, even a less important assignment, such as a cross training day, is a challenge for virtually every runner. Be brave, take the day off, and trust that come Saturday, you can execute a great long run.

What If I Were Paying Jay Johnson To Coach Me?

If you were paying me to coach you, you would listen to everything I communicated to you and 97% of the time you'd follow my instructions (with the remaining 3% of the time being a misunderstanding of what I communicated). The reason I share this is now that you own this book, you have the opportunity to adhere to the training laid out in the book as if I were your coach. I've shared everything I would ask you to do if you were a client, and you need to say to yourself, "This is basically the training I would get if I was paying $100 to $200 a month for coaching. If I follow the instructions and make the right choices throughout the training, I can run to my potential the way Jay's coached athletes do."

If you have several training books on your shelf, or you've been training with a group of runners for several years, then you have various ideas about training that are different than the principles in the SMT system. What you need to do now is fully invest in the SMT system. This is what clients that pay me do: they stop trying to combine several training plans into a plan that they think best fits them, and instead they follow my advice. I have no doubt that you'll have success if you do the same thing. You now know the SMT system, so it's time to work the system and run to your potential on race day.

In closing, there are many who will say that self-coached runners will never run to their potential. On one hand I agree with this statement, because I've seen so many runners make simple mistakes that lead to bad workouts, injury, and overtraining.

The SMT system isn't taking you to the edge of your physical capabilities in training. The SMT system intentionally includes ample recovery in the training schedule to absorb to inevitable times of excessive fatigue and illness. The point is, in the SMT system the chances of staying sick or having a string of bad workouts that lead to an injury is low. However, because there are choices and variables in the SMT system, making the right choice, day after day, is the key to running well as a self-coached runner.

If you are bit intimidated by the prospect of effectively following the SMT system I offer a semi-personal coaching plan that guides you through the SMT system. You'll get a weekly video, a daily email, guided audio workouts for the first three Tuesday workouts. Most important, you have the chance to ask me questions in a members only forum, a great way to ensure that you get the most out of your training.

Semi-Personal Coaching

For more information go to page 268 at the end of the book.

The bottom line is that you can coach yourself well so long as you are honest about how your body is feeling, how much life stress you have, and whether or not you can properly respond to the stress by altering your training for a day or two. Similarly, when you get the inevitable sickness during the 20-week cycle, you have to make the right choice and wait to run until you are 85-90% well. These are the things I tell coached clients in the midst of training. I'm telling you the same things, in advance, and giving you the responsibility to make the right call in real time.

TWEAKING THE SMT SYSTEM

"As to methods, there may be a million
and then some, but principles are few.
The man who grasps principles can
successfully select his own methods.
The man who tries methods, ignoring
principles, is sure to have trouble."

—Ralph Waldo Emerson

CHAPTER 14

Following The SMT System While Running Workouts And Long Runs On Different Days

If you lead a busy, hectic life, the best way to train for a marathon is simply to follow the SMT system 20-week cycle. That said, there are several ways that you can tweak the system to fit your individual needs as a runner and to make the system more enjoyable if you're someone who likes to race often.

If you are curious if you can run your workouts and long runs on days other than Tuesday and Saturday, the answer is yes, you absolutely can do this and still follow the SMT system. You simply need to shift the week forward or backward so that the rhythm of the week remains the same.

You could do Wednesday workouts and Sunday long runs; you could do Monday workouts and Friday long runs. You know the order of the days in the system, so you just have to shift your week. I've had clients run great marathons doing both the Wednesday/Sunday and Monday/Friday schedules, so by all means shift the schedule to make it fit your life.

If you do choose one of these alternate schedules, you need to get back to the normal SMT system schedule the week of the race. In chapter seventeen there are two 20-week training plans for both the Wednesday/Sunday and Monday/Friday schedules. These plans are unique in the lead-up to the 5k race in Week Four and they are different in the final two weeks of the 20-week cycle.

This is a great time to point out that I encourage you to run your long run on Sunday if there is a group of runners who regularly meet on Sunday for a long run. If you can meet a group for the long run on Sunday, I think it's a great opportunity that will benefit your training; even if they aren't doing the same run as you, you can at least start the run with other people. And who knows, maybe you can talk some of them into running your long run. Regardless, sharing a run with others is a joy. You do need to be careful that you execute your long run plan, which means that if you're not supposed to speed up until the final 3 miles of a run and the people around you are starting to accelerate, you must exert the discipline to hold back.

While there is a potential benefit to doing your long run on Sunday, what you cannot do is try to come up with a system where you run long on some Sundays and run long on some Saturdays. This alternation of long run days is not part of the SMT system. I don't need to go into detail to explain how the rhythm of the system is disturbed when you do this. Be smart and choose a long run day and stick to it.

Finally, if you choose to do your long run with others, you will probably be made fun of when you go straight from the long run into SAM work. Don't be surprised if people will tell you that you're training too hard, that you're wasting your time, that you're not recovering properly, etc. Ignore them and remind yourself that you are simply doing everything you can to become a better runner and to set yourself up for the best marathon you are capable of running.

Racing A Half Marathon During The 20-Week Training Cycle

Many runners will look at the SMT system 20-week training cycle and say, "I only get to race once and then I go for sixteen weeks without running another race? I usually race once every month or two, if not more. I don't know if I want to do this." My first response is that *if you want to do things you've never done before, then you have to do things you've never done before.* You've probably raced too often in the past and never given yourself the time to put in a solid block of training, a block of training that will result in better race performances than you've been getting by racing frequently.

That said, there is a way to run a race between the 5k in Week Four and the marathon in Week Twenty. You can race a half marathon during the 20-week training cycle, so long as you commit to follow the training laid out in the days following the race. Proper recovery from a half marathon race is critical. Many runners want to race, but they don't want to take time to recover. Make the right choice and follow the training that is laid out in the days after the race.

You will be racing, not simply running a controlled pace and finishing with plenty of energy in reserve. If you want to race the half marathon as part of an SMT system 20-week training cycle, then take the race seriously and run the best race you are capable of on that day. You won't be fully rested for the race, as you will have run a 12-mile long run the weekend before, yet the week of the race the volume of running is dramatically reduced, so you'll be able to run a solid performance.

Running a half marathon as part of a 20-week training cycle is not a bad idea and it's one that I encourage if you're someone who really likes to race.

That said, there are a two things you must do if you want to race well, weeks later, in the marathon. First, you need to have run 10 or 11 miles twice before you start the 20-week training cycle. The reason is simple: You will still need to safely progress your long runs so that you get in a 22-mile run before the marathon. The second thing you must do is trust the recovery days that follow the half marathon. Racing the half marathon takes one of your Saturday long runs away; running an easy run the weekend after your half marathon takes another Saturday long run away, as this is part of the recovery from the race. You need this much time to recover from the half marathon. The good news is that if you follow the training laid out in these two recovery weeks you will still be able to get in your 22-mile run in Week Sixteen of the 20-week training cycle.

The half marathon race comes in Week Thirteen of the training, seven weeks out from your marathon. Please don't try to alter the system and run a half marathon six weeks out or four weeks out from the marathon. I'm sure you've heard of people running half marathons this close to the marathon, but in the SMT system, where a large focus is the 22-mile run, you simply don't have enough time to race the half marathon and get in the 22-mile run. You've got to follow the SMT system and you've got to work the SMT system; running a half marathon at any week other than Week Thirteen is not part of the SMT system.

Note

Please refer to chapter seventeen for the 20-week training cycle that includes a half marathon in Week Thirteen. Remember, you have to have run 10 or 11 miles twice before you start this unique 20-week training cycle.

Travel Considerations When You Are Running An Out-Of-Town Race

If you are traveling to a race, be it an hour car ride from your home, or a flight across time zones, you need to make sure you are following the SMT system training in the days before the race. The key days before the race are the last four days of the training. Thursday is a day of complete rest, Friday is a 35-minute run with strides, Saturday is your pre-race day, and Sunday you race!

Let's look at the simple example first, where you are driving the day before the race, staying in a hotel the night before the race. You should set up your day so that you do leg swings before you get in the car to travel. When you arrive, you should do your pre-race routine, making sure to do leg swings at the end. I've said it before, and I'll say it again: Get in and out of the expo as efficiently as possible to minimize time on your feet the day before the race.

The same approach holds true for air travel. After you've been sitting for several hours on the plane, you want to make sure you do some leg swings before you get into the rental car, cab, or bus. Yes, you're going to look silly doing these, but you've worked so hard to get to this point that you don't want the last day or two before the race to go poorly because your legs/hips are tight and bound up.

Adjusting The SMT System Weekly Schedule Due To Work Travel

Business travel is stressful. When your life is stressful, you're not going to be training at 100%. Does this mean you can't train in the SMT system when you're traveling a great deal? No, but it does mean that if you make the right choices throughout the 20-week training cycle, there are a going to be a couple of times where you take a day off. Or, there may be a day or two where you have to shift the Tuesday workout to Wednesday, which is absolutely fine, though it will mean that you will skip the *tired legs run* altogether and get back on schedule with cross training on Thursday (I know, most of you hate this, but wisdom is the better part of valor).

If you're a business traveler, the biggest thing you need to do is acknowledge that you have a finite amount of energy. You're expending energy traveling, and, as is often the case, you're working longer hours when you're on a business trip than you do at home. Be honest with yourself about your energy levels and make the right choice with your training. You have to make a living, and if business travel is part of the equation, then you need to do the best job you can while you're traveling.

You can likely get in workouts and long runs when you're traveling, but you might have to run them slower than assigned. Or, you might be running low on energy and simply do an easy run with strides and SAM Easy. I can't tell you what to do in each situation, but I can tell you that if you take a moment to inventory how you're feeling, the right choice will be obvious. The right choice may not be what you want to do, e.g. run less, move the workout back a day, or take a day completely off. However, the right choice will usually be very clear.

QUESTION
&
ANSWER

"He who asks a question is a fool for five minutes; he who does not ask a question remains a fool forever."

— Chinese proverb

CHAPTER 15

Q: I just got this book and my marathon is coming up sooner than twenty weeks. Can I jump ahead a couple weeks and still do this program?

A: While you cannot jump into the SMT system if you don't have a full twenty weeks until your marathon, there are elements of the system that you can use in your training. First, the reason why you must not start the SMT system unless you have twenty weeks to do the entire program is simple: all of the elements of the system work together and will lose their effectiveness if truncated. Even if you are consistently running 12-mile runs before you read this book, you still can't start the training in Week Five (sixteen weeks to race day) because you would be four weeks behind in your journey of learning to run by feel and four weeks behind in the progression of SAM work. Both of these elements are critical to the system. If you are less than twenty weeks out from a marathon, simply be patient and follow a different training plan. Or, decide to run a half marathon rather than a marathon, and follow the SMT system for your next marathon. But the good news is that there are several elements that you can take from the book and use in your training immediately: Strides during your easy days, race pace work in the final five weeks of you training cycle, SAM work every day that you run. These three elements can be used in your marathon training immediately, and all three will positively impact your training.

Q: It doesn't make intuitive sense that the SAM Hard days come after workouts and long runs. Why are we doing it this way?

GEEK OUT
Read more about Concurrent Strength And Endurance Training on page 174

A: Go to the Geek Out section and read Dr. Carwyn Sharp's explanation of concurrent training and how that training is highly effective when done after your two challenging days of the week.

Q: Can I switch the order of the days if something comes up? For instance, on a given week, can I flip the Tuesday workout with the Wednesday tired legs run?

A: While you can't flip the days of these two runs, you can move your Tuesday workout to Wednesday. I would say this will probably need to happen at least once in the 20-week training cycle for the simple reason that you won't be fully ready to run a great Tuesday workout, due to sickness, or scheduling, or general life stress. In these cases, the best thing to do will be to move the Tuesday workout to Wednesday. If you make this switch in the week, you *do not* make up the Wednesday run on Thursday, but you get back on schedule and cross train on Thursday. This is *need to do,* not a *nice to do.* I know that you don't want to miss the Wednesday run, but that's just part of making the right choice when it comes to training in the SMT system. If you won't be 100% for a Tuesday workout, move it to Wednesday and get back on schedule by cross training on Thursday.

Q: Do I need a GPS watch or can I just use a normal watch?

A: I think there is a lot to be said for the GPS watch; my perspective is that it's a great investment in your running. It is helpful to have feedback during the last half of the 20-week training cycle when you are doing MP work. You need to groove MP and to do so you're going to need to check your watch every half-mile or mile for the first couple miles of a MP workout. Another reason to have a GPS watch is that it functions as a leash, keeping you from running too fast in the opening miles of race day. You can check your watch, without having to memorize splits, making sure you are running marathon pace and no faster. Finally, if you can find a watch that will beep when you hit a mile that is faster than the MP that you program into the watch, I would purchase that watch. My clients who have these watches and set the watch to beep when they go five seconds a mile too fast end up running better marathons because they are grooving the pace in the early miles of the race. One word of caution on the beeping aspect of these watches on race day: you probably don't want to set a "too slow" pace on your watch. Why? If you have a horrible day (which you probably will not) you don't want to be reminded that you're going slower than you had planned with a beeper that tells you that you are having a bad day. Just use the beep function on the watch to keep you from running too fast.

Q: Should I keep a training log? Should I keep my splits from each workout and long run? Should I keep my splits from easy runs?

A: Yes, you should keep a training log and you should note how you feel on each run. This information will be valuable when the marathon is over and you resume training for the next race. Over the course of several years you can see patterns in your training. While the SMT system keeps injuries to a minimum, training logs can be invaluable tools for going back and finding a pattern of training that leads to a certain type of injury or, conversely, a great performance. You definitely need to keep your splits from the Yasso 800s workout. You should keep the data from each long run and each MP workout as well. You don't necessarily need to keep the splits from the fartlek workouts, progression runs, and aerobic repeats, but many people do. Remember, you're running by feel in most of these workouts, so don't go into these workouts with an expectation about pace the first or second time you do one of these workouts. Please don't keep splits for your easy runs. Just trust the SMT system and run easy on your easy days. While you do have to get in the time assigned for these runs, along with strides, timing the run makes no sense when you consider that you're running by feel. If you have a set loop you do for your 55 minute easy run and you don't feel well one day, it's absolutely necessary that you run easy and let the run be 57 or 58 minutes. Running by feel will result in a few easy runs that will be slower than what you would normally run. No need to worry, this is by design.

Q: Why aren't there any hill workouts in the SMT system? I thought that I had to do some hill work to reach my potential.

A: Very good question. First, let's be clear that for all of your long runs that don't have MP running as part of the run, you are well served to run on a hilly course. Hill workouts aren't part of the SMT system for two reasons. The first is that every hill is different, e.g. a different grade and a different length. I can't create a system of training where there is variability for each athlete based on the topography that surrounds her. Second, hill workouts can easily become too intense and end up with the athlete producing significant amounts of lactate. If you're a miler that's fine, but if you're training for a marathon, you don't need or benefit from stressing the anaerobic system. Find a hilly course for your long runs if you can, yet trust that you don't need hill workouts in your training to run a great marathon.

Q: Should I be going to the weight room in addition to the SAM work?

A: No. SAM is plenty of work for you in your first SMT system 20-week training cycle. If you get to Phase 5 SAM in this training cycle, you should stay there for the rest of the 20-week cycle. You can visit *SimpleMarathonTraining.com* to watch videos that are the next progression of strength work. In your second 20-week cycle could use a medicine ball or kettlebell in addition to SAM. These two tools are great because you can keep them in your car, or keep them in your basement, and get a lot of great work done. But for the first 20-week cycle, just do SAM. You don't need to go to the weight room to gain the muscular strength and get the hormonal stimulus you need to keep improving as a runner. If you were a professional runner then there would be a couple of days per week that you would be in the weight room, but for the busy adult, leading a hectic life, there just isn't enough time. Trust SAM, and if Phase 5 isn't challenging you can visit *SimpleMarathonTraining.com* after the 20-week training cycle is over for guidance as to the next step in your strength work.

Q: I've been running marathon pace in workouts and long runs where marathon pace is assigned, but it feels hard and I don't know if I can do it on race day. Should I be worried?

A: No. Trust that the SMT system has empowered you to be able to run your goal MP for the entire 26.2 miles. Training is going to feel hard at times, especially before the taper begins. Even after the taper begins there are going to be times where MP doesn't feel easy, which you assume it would since you're only running MP for a few miles. You have to trust that all of the training will come together on race day and that you can run a great marathon when the gun goes off.

Q: I feel really good running marathon pace and I'm starting to think that my pace is too slow. Should I try to speed up?

A: No. Here's why: you will have a great experience running a marathon at a conservative pace, finishing strong in the last 6.2 miles of the race. If, at the end of the race, you finish saying, "I could have run faster!" that's a great outcome. Most runners who run race distances shorter than the marathon finish saying, "I know I could have run faster." Just run the MP that you've been grooving in your workouts and get to the 20-mile mark ready to grind. If you end up finishing knowing you could have run 1-2 minutes faster, that's still a great outcome, an outcome that will simply give you the motivation to train another twenty weeks (after your 4-week recovery cycle) so that you can run even faster.

Q: Why aren't there any prescribed down weeks in the training program?

A: That's a great question and I'll answer it three ways. First, my experience is that down weeks end up occurring as part of the program due to life stress or sickness that is not due to training. When you have a big project at work and need to take off both Wednesday and Thursday one week, that ends up making the week lighter in terms of training (though your life stress is high). Also, you need to understand that professional runners often have a down week because they are training at such high volumes and intensities. Professional marathoners train 120 miles or more a week, an intense amount of work that demands a down week for recovery. The SMT system never stresses your body to this extent, and you always have a chance to recover from a workout or a long run. Bottom line is, when you look back on your 20-week training cycle after completing your marathon, there will likely be a week where you trained fewer days with fewer minutes due to work related obligations or a sickness. Second, if you look at the five days leading up to the 22 mile run in Week Seventeen you'll see that each of these days is easier than what you've been doing. The Tuesday workout is the lightest workout you will have done in several weeks, and the duration of the days following it are all less than normal. While I wouldn't consider this a down week, there is no doubt that you're getting a bit of a respite in these five days from the volume and intensity of training you've been doing up to this point. Third, following the 22-mile run you A) walk briskly on Sunday B) take a day off on Monday, C) don't do a workout on Tuesday, but rather do an easy run with strides. Obviously three easy days in a row don't add up to a down week, but these are three more days that are easier than normal and will allow you to recover properly. Bottom line is that the 22-mile run is the single biggest day in the SMT system, so it only makes sense to rest up a bit before the run and properly recover following the run.

Q: Let's say I've gone through the 4-week recovery phase and my next goal is to run another marathon, yet that race is twenty-three weeks away. What should I do during the three weeks before the next SMT system 20-week cycle?

A: I would simply have fun with your running in the three weeks and make SAM the focus of your training. You don't want to try to train hard for twenty-three weeks, as this will likely be too challenging mentally. You might choose to run five days a week with a reasonable long run, but if you do, there is no reason to do workouts, though it's smart to do strides. Have the attitude that it is a great time to make progress with SAM work so that when the next SMT system 20-week cycle starts up, you can handle even more SAM work. The more SAM work you can handle, the faster you're going to run. Have fun with your running in these three weeks, and don't worry about doing any particular workouts or running a certain number of miles.

Q: Do you recommend I use a heart rate monitor?

A: Heart rate monitors have a place in running training. For the overtrained athlete who is resuming training, heart rate monitors can be used as a leash. The coach assigns a heart rate the athlete should not exceed while running. I personally used a heart rate monitor this way during a summer of college training and it worked very well. I would look at the watch and invariably late in the run I'd see that I was pushing up against the heart rate that I was trying to stay under. I took the cue and slowed down. You could argue that because of cardiac drift I should have continued running the pace I thought was easy. I disagree. I had overtrained the previous spring, which meant that I was running too hard on my easy days and not recovering. The summer was the time to learn this skill, and what better time to learn it than in the months when I was training on my own. In summary, heart rate monitors can be a useful tool when your goal is to keep from running too hard. The

GEEK OUT
Read more about Cardiac Drift on page 210

reason we won't be using heart rate monitors in the SMT system is that it's so easy to become a slave to your watch, interfering with the vital skill of running by feel.

Q: What shoes do I need? Do I need different shoes for long runs and workouts? What shoes should I race in?

A: This a good question and one that doesn't have a clear answer. While professional runners wear extremely lightweight shoes called racing flats when they race, for most runners it's going to make sense to simply wear the same shoe you've been using for your long runs. Why would you wear a heavier shoe in the race? Simple. You know the shoe that you've been in for hundreds of miles isn't going to cause you any problems. That said, you might want to consider buying a shoe that you can use for the long run and Tuesday workout that is a little lighter weight than the shoe you will wear on your easy days. Some people need a shoe that gives more support, and for the most part, supportive shoes are going to be a bit heavier. What does all of this equate to? Simply use the model of shoe that is working for you for most of your runs. If you are going to try a different shoe for the workouts and the long runs, then you need to do so at the start of the 20-week cycle, when the workouts are short and the long runs are short. The worst thing you can do is break in a new pair of shoes for a long run when you're running 16 miles or longer. Many a blister has formed under these circumstances. Final thought on footwear: Your fitness and muscular strength is going to get you to the finish line. Wear a shoe that won't cause you blisters or bloody toes. If your go-to shoe weighs a few ounces more than the lightweight shoe on the person next to you, so be it. You don't want to compromise twenty weeks of training by wearing a shoe that is going to cause you problems in the last 6.2 miles of the race.

Q: Can I run a half marathon and just run it for fun in the middle of the 20-week cycle?

A: No. Do the SMT system 20-week cycle, or choose the SMT system half marathon 20-week cycle, which allows you to race the half marathon as well as you can. Running one easy half marathon does nothing for you when you consider the following three issues. First, you could have run a long run that weekend, a run that would have been longer than 13 miles. Second, you'll have an extremely hard time not running the half marathon faster than that week's assigned long run. Third, you'll need to recover from the half marathon, even if you didn't race it, and this means you'll miss some good training, e.g. the Tuesday workout following the race. Final thought: in Week Five you have a

13-mile run; please heed my advice and don't run a half marathon that day, even though the race distance obviously fits the week's long run assignment.

Q: Can I run a half marathon as part of one of my long runs?

A: For many of the same reasons as I've pointed out above, trying to fuse a half marathon and a long run isn't a good idea. The first issue is that it's too easy to run too fast in this type of hybrid run. The second reason is that you likely won't have a good place to do your SAM work following the run. And the third reason is you won't be able to do a continuous run as you'll need to stand for a few minutes at the start of the race. So, let's say you wanted to do 5 miles and then hop in a half marathon. You'd have a few minutes after the initial 5 miles before you would be running again. The one reason it would make sense is to practice getting water and sports drinks during the race, but this isn't a compelling enough reason to try to combine a half marathon and a long run.

Q: I can't find a half marathon in Week Thirteen. Can I run it on a different week?

A: If you can't find a half marathon to run in Week Thirteen then you cannot run a half marathon as part of the SMT system. That's the right week to run a half marathon due to the recovery days you'll need following the race. If you try to run a half marathon later than the thirteenth week of the 20-week cycle then you'll run out of time to run your 22-mile long run. The good news is, you can simply follow the normal 20-week cycle and be ready to run a great marathon in Week Twenty.

Q: Can I qualify for Boston with this training program?

A: Absolutely. That said, you need to be close to a Boston qualifying time (BQ) before you start the 20-week cycle. It's realistic that if you follow the SMT system to the letter, you can run a 5 minute PR, though I can't guarantee a PR, as there are no guarantees in running. I want you to be honest about one issue if your goal is to qualify for Boston. You need to be process-oriented in your training and not outcome-oriented. Focus on becoming better every day, every week, every month. When you do so, you have a better shot

> **GEEK OUT**
> Read more about Growth Mindset on page 211

of reaching your goal of running a BQ time than if you just have that BQ time on the brain every time you head out for a run. It's great to have goals, but it's more important to focus on the process of staying injury-free, making the right choices in training, running by feel, and getting all of the SAM work done. These are the elements that will lead to a BQ time rather than a preoccupied focus on hitting a certain time.

Q: *I've qualified for Boston. Will this program get me ready for the race given that there is no hill training in the SMT system?*

A: Great question. There isn't a clear-cut answer to this one. On one hand, Boston is a 26.2-mile race that requires you to be fit and to be able to utilize fat as an energy source. The SMT system will get you fit and teach your body to utilize fat as an energy source. These are the fundamentals of running a marathon well, and obviously the SMT system can help you with those two goals. The ideal Boston Marathon training plan would have some running on long downhills and then have you learn to run well after having beat up your legs a bit. Most runners will have more confidence on Heartbreak Hill having done some hill workouts, even though I've made a compelling argument that hill workouts aren't necessary in marathon training (and Heartbreak Hill is in fact quite short). The biggest factor that you need to be honest about when you train for Boston is that if you live in a flat area and don't have a hilly long run course, you're going to be at a bit of a disadvantage. The converse is that if you have qualified for Boston and live in a hilly area, then you are doing yourself a disservice if you don't go out and run most of your long runs on those hilly courses. Simply put, if you want to run a somewhat hilly marathon well, you should do hilly long runs to prepare.

Q: *Why do you take off Thursday before a Sunday race in the SMT system?*

A: Taking a full day of rest in advance of the marathon—meaning no running or cross training—is a great way to feel fresh and energetic on race day. You definitely don't want to take the day off before the race (which you probably knew before reading this book). For many years I was a proponent of taking a day off on Friday before a Sunday race. However, what I've found is that athletes tend to be antsy in anticipation for the race. A Friday run helps them deal with their antsiness by expending some energy. Taking the day off with a bit more lead time (Thursday), when the nerves aren't as great, allows you to get the rest in and also deal with your nervous energy through running in the couple days before the race. If you must do something on the rest day, you can do a bit of AIF. Or, you can walk in the pool for 10 minutes, or do some hip mobility (not hip strengthening) exercises from SAM Easy. You can and should go through your imagery routine on this day, as you're just a few days away from the race.

Q: Why aren't there any threshold runs or tempo runs in the SMT system?

A: First, I want to acknowledge all of the research that shows that running near your threshold or just under your threshold produces great aerobic gains. The reason the workouts on Tuesday tend to be a little longer than a threshold run, but done a little slower than a typical threshold run, is that we want to take advantage of the one day a week where you have more time to train. As you read previously, there will be quite a bit of MP running in the final weeks of the training. Prior to this, you will do workouts like progression runs, some 50 and 60 minutes in duration, and these are great aerobic workouts. The biggest reason I don't prescribe threshold runs or tempo runs is that doing so would force me to assign you a time for the run. What if you slept horribly the night before, or have a big work deadline that is causing anxiety, or you are dealing with a sick child? In the SMT system, you can show up on Tuesday morning and feel good about the workout if you simply complete it along with your SAM Hard. Too often, when you are assigned a pace for a workout, e.g., threshold pace or tempo pace, you have to run harder than you should to hit the pace. You're not running a threshold workout as much as you're hanging on, running an effort that is well past challenging and closer to a race effort (or survival effort). The SMT system works, and I promise that if you go through the 20-week cycle and learn to run by feel, you will make great aerobic gains.

Q: What if I simply can't run the Yasso workouts well. Can I still run a good marathon?

A: Every once in a while I work with a client who really struggles to do the Yasso workout, even if the other workouts and long runs are going well. The first thing to understand about this workout is that it should be done on a track.

Some runners dislike running on the track and the thought of doing close to thirty laps for a workout sounds horrible. If you fall into this category, my advice is simple: Do your best to remember that there are only three days in the 20-week training cycle (three days out of one hundred and forty) that you are assigned the Yasso workout. You've committed to running a great marathon and doing these workouts well is simply part of the process of being able to run a great marathon. Once you've committed to running the Yasso workout as well as you can, there is still the possibility of not performing well. The importance of the Yasso 800s workout is that you need it to gauge your fitness in the SMT system and to come up with a reasonable MP for both the training in the last few weeks of the 20-week cycle and for race day. Having a reasonably accurate MP pace is important. Using an MP for training and the race that is faster than your level of fitness will set you up for unnecessary suffering when you pass the 20-mile mark in the race and are forced to do the painful shuffle of a runner who has started the race too fast. Arriving at 20 miles feeling great and able to speed up just a tiny bit in the last 6.2 miles of the race is much preferable and is the goal of the SMT system. If the weather forecast for the Yasso 800s workout is poor, you should go inside and run the workout on the treadmill. Set the treadmill to a 1-2% grade and then do the workout. After the workout, you should add 2-3 seconds per 800m to your time as most people run faster on the treadmill than they would outdoors. If you end up running the workout in wind/rain/snow, you can assume that you would have run your Yasso workout a bit faster, so take off 1-2 seconds per 800m when you calculate your average 800m time for the workout. Finally, this is one of the areas in the 20-week training cycle where you might benefit from the *SimpleMarathonTraining. com* semi-personal coaching, as you would be able to ask questions about your workout in the forum.

Q: I've seen other training programs that say to take a complete day off once a week. Should I do the same and skip either the Thursday cross training day or the brisk walk on Sunday?

A: That's a great question, and there are two ways to look at it. The first way is that we want to follow the mantra of *when in doubt, do less*. With this in mind, it absolutely makes sense to take Thursday off if you think that's what you need do to train at a high level. You don't want to take off Sunday because the way you're going to recover from a challenging long run is doing the brisk walk. Thursday is a day where you're not gaining fitness, but rather maintaining fitness, so taking the day off is reasonable. My one caution against taking a day off each week is that you must remember that you're only running five days a week in the SMT system. While I can't quantify the positive or negative impact of taking Thursday completely off, I do know that when people learn the system, trust the system, and work the system, they run well. With this in mind, I suggest you follow the system.

Q: Is there anything I should do differently for my next marathon after having completed the SMT system for one marathon? For instance, should I run more miles, do more SAM work, do different workouts?

A: This is a great question. The simple answer is that if you've done the SMT system once and had success, there is a very good chance that repeating the system for a second marathon will result in running even faster. Most of the best runners in the world do not change their workouts and long run assignments for each marathon cycle, but rather keep the same workouts and long runs in place, with the goal of running just a touch faster. You should do the same for your second marathon in the SMT system. After going through the SMT system twice, you can argue that you can handle a bit more training, but only if your schedule and your life stress allows for it. You should definitely plan to move through the next phases of SAM. If you get to Phase 5 SAM and you can do so without issue, then you can add additional strength work, such as kettlebell training.

Q: My race is on Saturday and not Sunday. How do I adjust the schedule in the final two weeks of the 20-week training cycle to account for this?

A: In chapter seventeen there is a two week training cycle for a Saturday race. This simple schedule will have you rested and ready to go on race day.

Q: Why can't I switch days? For instance, why can't I do my tired legs run *on Tuesday and then my workout on Wednesday?*

A: This is a bad idea. Why would you want to go into a workout having run a longer run the day before? Plus, remember that your body will have adapted to doing strides the day before a workout, which allows the workout to feel easier. Even if you keep the run on Tuesday easy, just as you would with a Wednesday run, you'll be flat for your workout on Wednesday. You must trust the rhythm of the week. Changing the rhythm means you're not following the SMT system and therefore you can't expect the same results as those who follow the system.

Q: If I have to move my Tuesday workout to Wednesday, why can't I do the tired legs run *on Thursday rather than cross train?*

A: In the SMT system you never run more than three days in a row. Could you run four or five days in a row? Probably, yet the chance of injury for a busy adult goes up when you try to run that many days without a break. In the scenario you're suggesting, you run Wednesday, Thursday, Friday, and Saturday—four days in a row. More importantly, you have two harder days, a workout on Wednesday and *tired legs run* on Thursday, and then go right into a Friday run. This means that you've had harder days two out of the three days prior to the most important workout of the week, the long run. If you've been following the SMT system, there is a very good chance that you will feel fatigued and have a long run that doesn't go well if you decide to deviate from the SMT system. Again, trust the system and trust that if you have to move your Tuesday workout to Wednesday, the right choice is to get back on track Thursday for the cross training day.

Q: How do I deal with an injury in the SMT system?

A: This is a common question, and unfortunately there is no single correct answer. First, you need to find a health care practitioner who works with runners and can properly diagnose the injury. You need to do the research and find someone who works with runners on a regular basis. For instance, there may be a great physical therapist in your town who works with geriatric patients. This physical therapist is probably not the practitioner for you.

GEEK OUT
Read more about Finding A Practitioner on page 192

It's impossible to address all of the various injuries that runners deal with; what I can say, after twenty five years of training and coaching, is that taking a day or two off is rarely a bad idea. A day or two of rest to decrease significant stress will help the body heal. Take this a step further and find a practitioner who can give you rehabilitation exercises and modalities to help you organically let your body recover. The final point to make about injuries is that if you take care of them, you can be running again without too much delay. The problem is that you won't be able to go back into the SMT 20-week training cycle where you might like, but instead have to enter the training cycle at the point where you last left off. This is where maturity and having the long view of your running career is important. You may not be able to run the goal marathon time you had hoped to run, yet you can run a solid marathon and finish the race injury-free. Many (most?) runners finish a marathon with some sort of injury and have to take weeks off after the race before they can train again. *This doesn't need to be you!* Address your injury and resume training where you left off in the 20-week cycle and arrive at the starting line of the marathon injury-free.

GEEK OUT

"Learning never exhausts the mind."

— Leonardo da Vinci

CHAPTER 16

Your Long Run
Carwyn Sharp, PhD

For decades, and arguably over a century, the long run has been foundational to the training of middle and long distance runners. Iconic coaches such as Sir Arthur Lydiard, Dr. Jack Daniels, and many others, as well as world and Olympic champions, all talk about the important role of long aerobic runs in developing and maintaining the physiological and psychological characteristics necessary for competitive and recreational athletes.

More recently, exercise scientists, coaches, and athletes have been delving deeper into the specific programming aspects of this training tool to determine how to further optimize the adaptive effects of the long run. For example, how long is long enough if you're an elite versus recreational runner? What's the optimal intensity if you're aiming for a 3:30 or Olympic qualifying time? Should you do a long aerobic run once a week or every other week?

While some questions have yet to be answered, what we do know is that the positive adaptations we see from chronic aerobic endurance training programs are the result of the additive effects of each single training session. These additive effects and subsequent adaptation are specific to the types of stresses these sessions place on the body. This is what is meant by the term "specificity of training." Stress is a key concept underpinning all the positive changes we experience when we train. The body will only change and adapt if you place it under more stress than it normally encounters. Running longer distances and higher intensities than your body is accustomed to will place sufficient stress on the body to cause it to adapt further than its current state. Getting outside your comfort zone is important if you want to improve your race results. This was originally described by a Canadian endocrinologist, Hans Selye, who was studying the roles of the adrenal gland and stress hormones in adapting to stress and sickness. He called this process of stress and adaptation the General Adaptation Syndrome.

Now, let's look at the long run from a physiological perspective, to examine how it stresses the body's tissues and systems, and what positive adaptations occur in the recovery afterwards.

First of all, *fuel*. There's no doubt that 26.2 miles is a long way to run and will require a lot of fuel or energy, regardless of what time you are aiming to run. As Jay has discussed, it's reasonable to assume it will require the average runner 2,500+ kcal to run a marathon. And yet, we store only approximately 1,800 kcal of carbohydrates (in the form of glycogen) in our muscles and liver, and glucose in our blood. Running long stresses the ability of this relatively limited amount of stored carbohydrate to meet the demands of prolonged endurance exercise such as running a marathon.

Depleting or significantly reducing your muscle and liver glycogen stores has two advantageous long-term adaptations. Firstly, *super-compensated glycogen stores*.[1] Glycogen is the large branched storage form of carbohydrate, somewhat like a tree structure with the branches representing a form of glucose. The branching structure increases the surface area of the glycogen so it is more easily and rapidly broken down to make the glucose more readily available when you need it. Long runs significantly reduce or deplete your glycogen stores and stimulate your muscles to store more glycogen than they did previously. This is great news, because increasing our glycogen stores means we need to consume less during the marathon (which can cause some people GI distress). It is worth noting that muscle biopsy data also shows that exercise sessions that do not significantly reduce your fuel stores appear to have little effect on increasing glycogen above initial levels.

This leads to the next physiological reason why including long runs in your marathon training is a good idea. You burn more fat![2] Scientifically it's more accurate to say that long runs stimulate the body to use more fat and less glycogen (glycogen sparing), but I prefer hearing I'm burning more fat than sparing glycogen. Considering we have such limited stores of glycogen, using a higher percentage of fat for fuel at a given speed or intensity is obviously a good thing and will help us all to run farther. Even though our bodies are using more fat, at low to moderate intensity, fat typically only accounts for 50 or 60% of the total fuel source. The adage often used by exercise physiologists is "fat burns in a carbohydrate flame." In order for your muscles to use fat as a fuel source, carbohydrates must be available and used at the same time.

What does all this mean? It means that by completing long runs regularly throughout your training program, you not only increase your fuel stores of glycogen, but you also reduce the amount of glycogen you will be using by increasing the amount of fat used instead, which ultimately means we've reduced the risk of "hitting the wall" in other words, becoming   glycogen depleted.[3]

To explain this more deeply, with chronic aerobic endurance training sessions we see an *increase in both the number and size of mitochondria in trained muscles*.[4] Mitochondria are specialized structures or compartments within muscle cells (and other types) which perform a variety of different functions, but perhaps most important to distance runners is that mitochondria convert energy from macronutrients in food into energy that the cell can use, called ATP (adenosine triphosphate). It's these little aerobic power plants that allow muscle cells to burn more fat and less glycogen. In terms of running performance, this adaptation means you are able to maintain a faster pace while remaining aerobic physiologically.

Use it or lose it! While it only takes a few weeks to see a measurable improvement in mitochondrial density of muscle with the stimulus of aerobic training sessions, unfortunately, approximately 50% of these gains can be lost in as little as one week of not training.[5] The moral of this story is that consistency of training is critical!

Another muscular adaptation you can expect, but may not be able to see (unless we do a muscle biopsy!), is an *increase in the activity of the aerobic enzymes* within your mitochondria responsible for aerobic energy production.[6] Not only is there an increase in the number of these aerobic enzymes due to an increase in the number and size of the mitochondria in which they reside, but in conjunction they become more active; the mitochondria are more efficient at aerobic metabolism.

Your skeletal muscle cells change in other ways as well. While it appears from the latest research that the proportion of slow twitch (aerobic) and fast twitch (anaerobic) muscle fibers/cells you have is genetically predetermined, with elite marathoners having as much as 90% slow twitch, aerobic long runs cause the fast twitch fibers to become more like slow twitch fibers. That's because there are actually hybrid fibers that exist on a continuum between the two "pure" fibers.

Aerobic training causes the fast twitch fibers to move on the continuum to be more like slow twitch within the fast twitch realm.[7] These hybrids are more aerobic and fatigue-resistant than fast twitch and so support the long-distance athlete more than the anaerobic fast twitch athlete.

The cardiovascular system also undergoes significant positive changes with recurring aerobic training sessions.

Regular long runs typically expose us to prolonged but varying levels of heat and dehydration. Quite often the rate at which we sweat is greater than our ability to consume and absorb water and electrolytes. As a consequence, throughout the duration of the long run we become progressively more dehydrated. To avoid serious medical complications you should aim to not lose more than 2-3% of your body weight during any exercise bout. With these repeated prolonged exposures our blood volume increases as a product of an increase in red blood cells and plasma (the fluid part of blood).[8] An increase in the number of red blood cells allows for more oxygen to be carried from the lungs to the working tissues, and also for more carbon dioxide, and indirectly more hydrogen ions from lactic acid, to be transported back to the lungs and removed from the body. Greater amounts of plasma mean we are better able to cope with heat and loss of sweat because we have a larger reservoir of fluid in our body to draw from.

The number of capillaries which surround each muscle fiber/cell also increases.[9] This results in an increased ability to deliver oxygen, fuel, water, and nutrients to the working muscles, and also to remove metabolites such as lactate and carbon dioxide along with various metabolic waste products.

Delivery of more oxygen to our muscles won't improve performance unless the oxygen can get into the cell and then to the mitochondria where it can ensure aerobic metabolism continues. This transport of oxygen within the muscle cell is the role of myoglobin, a protein similar to the hemoglobin which binds oxygen to red blood cells for transport in the blood. Repeated long runs *increase myoglobin levels,* allowing more oxygen to be transported within the cell and consequently increasing the aerobic capacity of the cells.[10]

While the focus of this Geek Out is the physiological adaptations, don't underestimate the powerful psychological benefits to the long run. Long runs add confidence in knowing you can run on tired legs for 20+ miles—as most people do their long run on the weekend, the fatigue from the training earlier in the week isn't fully dissipated. And, when things don't quite go according to plan on of these long runs (you forget your anti-chafe product! or you feel the accumulating fatigue making your legs heavy), you have the knowledge that you can overcome them during the race, just like you did in training.

So, if the aerobic long runs are so beneficial, how long is long enough? Even though the research on the physiological effects of aerobic training on endurance performance has been ongoing for many decades, there is no definitive scientific research that answers this question. There is scientific evidence to show that longer durations result in greater gains in muscle mitochondrial density.[11] But, because this isn't a linear relationship, there is undoubtedly a point at which going longer will not result in a further increase in mitochondria. Don't forget that running long results in many other positive adaptations. While diminishing returns can come into play for some aspects of your fitness when running longer than 90 minutes, many other factors may continue to show improvements.

The adaptive effects of training duration are coupled to those of intensity. Higher intensities of training elicit mitochondrial improvements with shorter duration.[12] While this can seem attractive from a time management standpoint, and there certainly is a place for higher intensity training sessions, replacing longer aerobic sessions with high intensity has been speculated to result in a decline in adaptations in slow twitch fibers (increased mitochondria with high intensities results in adaptations in fast twitch fibers) and a possible decline in endurance performance. Only short, high intensity training would also likely negate the glycogen sparing, cardiovascular, and other aerobic adaptations.

Finally, the key to getting the maximum benefit out of your long runs is to be well prepared for them by gradually and appropriately building up the distance, and also allowing sufficient time afterwards to recover. Train smarter, not harder, and reap the rewards!

Concurrent Strength and Endurance Training
Carwyn Sharp, PhD

As a parent or busy professional (or both!), it can be difficult to find the time to train. The idea of combining strength training and running into one workout can be attractive so you don't have to leave the house or office twice to work out. Combining endurance and strength training one after the other in a single session is called concurrent training.

Popular belief used to be that because strength training leads to increases in muscle mass and strength, whereas endurance training tends to cause a net catabolic state (breakdown of muscle) resulting in a loss of mass and improved aerobic capacity, these modes of training were incompatible. The hormonal responses to these modes of training are also different, and are some of the prime drivers of adaptation and recovery or breakdown. Running is a stressful endeavor and so it is not surprising that secretions of the stress hormone cortisol increase in response.

Aerobic training, especially running, is often associated with an increase in net protein breakdown (catabolism) of skeletal muscle, due to a number of factors, including increased levels of cortisol and other stress hormones in the blood.[1,2] Anabolic (tissue-building) hormones such as testosterone, growth hormone and insulin-like growth factor-1 (IGF-1) also increase with endurance exercise, although typically not to the same extent as the catabolic, resulting in an overall catabolic state.[3] It's not all bad news! The better trained you are, the faster you adapt to these hormonal responses, *and* the anabolic response increases more. Other research that supports this is the finding that in the skeletal muscle of endurance-trained athletes, net protein synthesis (anabolic is greater than catabolic), which is most likely due to mitochondrial rather than contractile proteins.[4,5]

Early research supported the contention that resistance training may cause a reduction in endurance capacity by decreasing mitochondrial density in muscle cells.[6] Later studies found that concurrent strength and endurance training did not appear to reduce endurance performance, and others suggested strength training combined with endurance training may actually improve endurance performance and various physiological measures associated with endurance performance such as VO^2max and lactate threshold.[7,8,9,10,11] Even more recently, it has been shown that certain strength training programs can actually increase mitochondrial density.[12]

So what explains the contradictions in the research? It appears that at least part of the explanation is the kind of strength training that is undertaken. Several studies have shown that more sport-specific explosive resistance training with lighter resistance, when combined with aerobic training, resulted in improved running economy and performance (3,000m and 5,000m).[13] When highly trained runners utilize concurrent endurance, resistance, and plyometric training (using only body weight), researchers see significant improvements in peak running velocity and 3,000m time trial compared to endurance training alone.[14]

Adding resistance training on top of an existing endurance training program risks overtraining; some scientists have postulated that this may be why some concurrent research has failed to show improvements in performance.[15,16] For example, when resistance and endurance training was alternated for 6 days, the results were impaired, but when both types of training were combined into one session, allowing a day of recovery in between workouts, more favorable results were found.[17,18,19] Another approach has been to replace running with explosive strength training and body weight plyometrics so the total training time, or energy expenditure, isn't increased, and thus the risk of overtraining is mitigated. One group had elite distance runners decrease their running by 32% and instead participate in explosive strength training and plyometrics.[20] When compared to running alone, this program significantly improved the athletes' 5,000m times.

The bottom line is that concurrent strength and endurance training, applied in an appropriately progressive and periodized manner, can actually increase one's endurance performance. The key is to utilize explosive-type exercises, and to be prudent with recovery.

Should You Run When You Are Sick?
Jay Johnson, MS

At some point in the training, you're likely to get sick. The question becomes, should you run when you're sick?

The simple answer is no, though I know this is not what you want to hear. You love running, you love being active, and to have this taken away, if only for a day, can be extremely frustrating. The more subtle answer is that you can run when you are 85-90% well. That's the threshold (obviously a subjective one) that you need to be honest about when you decide to resume running again.

For me, consistency is the concept I think of when an athlete gets sick or has a cold. My job as a coach is to have them take as few days off as possible. What most runners without a coach do is keep training while sick, which often means that it takes them five to seven days to feel well. I would rather an athlete take two days completely off and see if they can get to feeling 85-90% well. If they can, then on the third, fourth, or fifth day they can go for an easy 35-minute run. A couple of days of easy running and you can get back on the 20-week training cycle.

When you do an easy run with strides on a day that you are coming back from sickness, you will likely feel close to 100% in the first few hours after your run. Don't trust this window of time as the accurate measurement of where you are and where you will be when you wake up. Feeling 100% after your first run back is common, but feeling and being 100% the next morning is not common. When you wake up the next morning, take inventory of how you feel and use the 85-90% rule to decide if you should go for a run or not.

When it comes to doing a Tuesday workout, a Wednesday *tired legs run* or the Saturday long run, you should be feeling 100%. So, if you wake up Tuesday and are at 90%, you need to have the courage and discipline to run an easy 35-45 minutes and strides, hoping that you are ready to go Wednesday morning. Another example would be to wake up Friday and feel 90%, which means you do your normal easy run with strides. Unfortunately you wake up Saturday feeling no better. You should not run the long run, but rather replicate Friday and set yourself up for feeling 100% by Monday.

It's important that I point out that you will have others (friends, coaches, running partners) telling you that you can train through a cold, but not the flu. For me, the answer to this issue is simple, and it comes back to consistency. My experience is that the athletes who take complete days off and rest when they are sick, are sick for fewer days, which means that they get the chance to run workouts and long runs sooner than if they had gutted it out for five to seven days, running at less than 80% of their capacity. As I explained above, if you miss a couple of days but are ready to resume workouts after three, four, or five days, you're now back on track for your normal training load.

The final question you should be asking yourself is, "Do I keep following the 20-week training cycle, or do I need to go back and do the workouts or long runs that I missed?" Good question.

If you missed a Yasso workout in Week Fourteen, then you need to make up this workout. For everything else, you should simply move your training back a week and remember that most people will miss some part of the 20-week cycle, so it's not the end of the world if you have to miss a couple of days. If you end up missing a long run, you should be able to get back on the schedule. For example, if you missed the 16-mile run in Week Nine, then you need to do 16-miles in Week Ten, rather than the 18 miles that is assigned. This allows you to do an 18-mile run in Week Eleven, which asks you to run 18 miles and speed up at the end if you feel well. I hope this doesn't sound complicated because in actuality it's not. If you do get sick, remember the mantra *make the right choice*. It will help you slow down, thoughtfully consider, and make the right choice!

The rule with illness and colds is simple. You have to be 85-90% well to run, and you have to be 99% well to do workouts and long runs.

Active Isolated Flexibility
AIF, aka "rope stretching"
Doug Petrick
Busy Father, Teacher and Coach

I started using AIF routines about three years ago after I sustained a running injury (stress fracture and ankle tendon damage) that put me on the shelf for the better part of nine months. Please note, the injury was incurred before Coach Jay and I began working together.

I reached out to Jay via email about ancillary work that I could perform that would make me "feel like a runner" during the recovery period. Mentally and physically, I knew it would be a challenge to deal with time away from running. I derive a lot of joy from the routine of training and racing. Luckily, Jay recommended Phil Wharton's Active Isolated Flexibility (AIF) and Active Isolated Strength (AIS) routines as work that I could incorporate into my recovery routine. Additionally, he stressed that AIF and AIS work are items that I should continue to devote time to once I was ready to start running again.

Upon his recommendation, I purchased Phil Wharton's Active Isolated Flexibility and Strength for Runners DVD/Stretch Rope package. I listened to a few interviews with Phil Wharton to get better insight into how and why this work was important for runners of all ability levels. It was a revelation to hear him describe elite athletes that had struggled with similar issues and took steps to break the injury cycle. The routine of AIF and AIS was the common thread for these elite runners to stay healthy, injury-free, and consistent with their training. As a result, these runners were able to use consistent training to reach PRs and increase their training workloads.

I am not an elite runner, but I am a busy adult, like most runners. We all have different facets of our life that we enjoy and manage: family, work, school, training, etc., all things that contribute to spreading us thin.

Thus, time is always a limiting factor for busy adult runners. Before you commit to the AIF work, you have to trust that 10-15 minutes a day is a sound investment in order to make you a better runner. It didn't take much time for me to buy into the AIF work. Prior to using AIF as a part of my daily routine, I was not able to string together large training blocks. Before investing in AIF work, I would improve for weeks, incur a minor injury, take off time from running, then start from ground zero.

The tradeoff for AIF and Active Isolated Strengthening (AIS) just makes so much sense. Carving out 10-15 minutes a day for AIF and AIS has kept me healthy and injury-free as a runner.

The way that I've been able to successfully incorporate AIF & AIS into my daily routine is to make it a part of my "powering down" night time ritual. I am married, run, teach, coach, and have three young kids. I've made AIF a part of the nighttime routine when I put the children to bed. I keep a Wharton Stretch Rope under my bed and after tucking the kids in, I move through the "10-minute quick release AIF routine." The AIF & AIS routines work great as a relaxation exercises. Depending on the schedule for the day, sometimes the AIF & AIS routines are used directly before running as a warm-up or directly after running as a cool-down. However, no matter what the day brings, I always look forward to the time I've carved out for the AIF and AIS work before I go to bed. Once your body becomes accustomed to the movements, you will feel physically centered and stronger. You'll also get a sense of relaxation from the work you're performing—knowing it will improve your training as a busy adult runner.

I also use the "foot/ankle quick release AIF routine" multiple times a day based upon how my foot feels. I always perform it at night typically right before the total body AIF routine. If my foot/ankle mobility feels limited, I will do the foot/ankle AIF routine in the morning when I am getting ready for work and throughout the day as needed. Even though my injuries have healed, I've made the AIF & AIS routines an integral part of my training. On days that I don't run or train, the AIF and AIS are the constant.

I've found that AIF and AIS has allowed me to improve as a runner, but I've had to commit to doing this work. One of the keys is for a runner to understand the importance of non-running work and how it will allow you to become a better runner. AIF and AIS has allowed me to break the cycle of injury. As a result, I've been able to string together large blocks of training.

As a runner, I've never felt stronger and more in tune with my body. The investment of performing AIF and AIS work has made me feel physically and mentally centered. The cumulative effect is that I've run faster times in races, increased the intensity of my training, and increased my strength, mobility, and flexibility.

The Importance of Strength and Mobility
Alia Gray, Professiional Runner
Marathon PR of 2:34:00

I have always loved the concept of strength work outside of my running. Getting stronger—sounds like a great idea, right? However, until my professional career really got underway, I didn't have a full routine written specifically for my type of training cycle. I'd walk into the gym and create a small smorgasbord of what I felt like was probably getting the job done.

Forging ahead with little to no structured plan is not a good way to set yourself up for success. I would never go blindly into my running workouts without having a grasp on why certain workouts are being implemented and what kind of fitness gains I'm looking to build from. Why should strength work be any different?

In general, runners across the board want to do the running work, but are uncertain of where to begin when it comes to the ancillary work, which makes it easier to just not do it. Other runners are a little phobic of strength work, worried that it may make them bulk up and add unwanted muscle mass. Rest assured, when you're doing the right type of strength work, this really shouldn't be a problem.

I work in Strength and Mobility daily—some days are a little more involved than others, but the key aspect of it, just like running, is consistency. As I rack up the years as a distance runner, it becomes more and more difficult to ignore the necessity of strength and mobility work. As runners, we get pretty darn good at moving in one plane of motion – forward. I realize when I do ancillary work how neglected every other aspect of movement can become if running is the only form of exercise.

Do you know what the really great thing about ancillary work is? If you work on the other aspects and planes of movement it will actually make you faster, healthier, more athletic, and more efficient in the forward running movement plane that we love so much.

I have dedicated a larger portion of my life to the pursuit of this sport than most people, but I still have to remind myself to be consistent about my strength work. There are days when the hours seem to compress on themselves, work deadlines come sooner than expected, and in general it seems impossible to get the day's tasks accomplished. I somehow manage to get my run in, but if anything is going to be cut, strength work is the first to go.

What I've learned is, don't cut the strength work! Doing at least some of the strength and mobility work doesn't take too long; instead of cutting these routines completely, maybe shave off a couple miles of running in order to sneak in some strength work—it's that important.

Since I've begun doing a regimen of ancillary routines, the few times that I've gotten in a rut of neglecting strength and mobility due to time constraints, I start to feel little nagging issues begin to pop up: a kneecap that feels a little tweaked, or a hip flexor that's too tight. These sorts of nags are not great for maintaining a consistent running routine. It is far better to cut a couple miles here or there in order to maintain the strengthening and mobility work.

I'll end by sharing with you a little personal tip: I really like my mobility routines as a meditative exercise just before bed. I keep myself pretty busy throughout the week and sometimes have a difficult time completely powering down my mind for sleep. Lying on the ground, slowly and intentionally going through my daily hip mobility routine provides a bit of a cathartic release.

You Do Hard Things
Cindy Kuzma, Freelance Writer
Contributing Editor to
Runner's World

Y ou can do it!" "You're strong." "You can accomplish anything you set your mind to." From childhood, most of us hear these types of encouraging phrases from parents, teachers, coaches, and teammates.

Research suggests you can use self-talk to channel the positive energy they create—and you might want to do it verbatim. In one study in the *European Journal of Social Psychology*, college students were more likely to follow through on their intentions and also did better on a difficult problem-solving task when they spoke or wrote down encouraging statements that began with "you" instead of "I."

The study authors, from the University of Illinois and University of Pennsylvania, posit that talking to yourself in the second person more effectively conjures words from others than if you were to use first-person language. When your subconscious believes you have a team behind you, you'll naturally view stressful situations as challenges instead of threats.

In my own training, I've found it helpful to combine this technique with a dash of realism—something I learned from Chicago dietitian and behavior change expert Dawn Jackson Blatner, R.D.N. Platitudes like *"You're feeling strong!"* or *"You got this!"* ring hollow when I'm struggling or fearing the discomfort ahead in a workout or race. Instead of focusing on beliefs about my ability or resolve, which my brain can all too easily discount, I find it more meaningful to acknowledge the facts: This situation, be it the last 5 minutes of a progression run or the last 6.2 miles of a marathon, is definitely difficult. But that's why I signed up, and I'm up to the challenge.

So my mantra of choice? "You do hard things." When I repeat this, I'm reminded that not everyone chooses to log 22 miles on a hilly route, run 800-meter repeats into driving wind and rain, or hit the gym to do 25 minutes of strength-training after an hour-long fartlek workout. I do hard things all the time, and this time will be no exception. In a way, it's like having Jay, my husband Matt, or another supportive fan there on the sidelines, reassuring me I have what it takes to push through and prevail.

The Latest Sleep Science
Carwyn Sharp, PhD

We have all experienced how a poor night of sleep, or insufficient sleep, can negatively affect our ability to think and function at normal levels. However, a Finnish study shows 20% of individuals suffer from chronic insufficient sleep, defined as losing 1 hour or more of sleep at night than is needed (7.5 to 9 hours of sleep per night is recommended).[1] A Harvard Medical School study (2007) suggests as many as 60% of women may be sleep deprived. Surprisingly, it has also been shown that sleep insufficiency is relatively common in elite athletes as well.[2] If the increasing sales of coffee (specialty coffee sales are increasing 20% per year) and energy drinks (sales topped $9 billion in 2015) in the U.S. are anything to go by, it seems we *really* like our caffeine, and many may feel they need it!

So, why should we care if we're not getting the recommended amount of sleep? While no one has been able to definitely show why the brain and body need to sleep, nonetheless, sleep is arguably the most important tool for recovery that we have. Understanding how sleep affects recovery provides opportunities to maximize recovery. The recovery aspects of sleep are largely mediated through the endocrine (hormonal) system.[3] Melatonin is a key hormone involved in sleep and is primarily secreted by the pineal gland in the brain. Melatonin levels increase in the late afternoon/evening as darkness approaches and decrease in the early morning as it gets closer to dawn. Melatonin acts and facilitates significant actions as an anti-inflammatory and antioxidant agent and facilitator.[4] Melatonin is also a positive modulator of the immune system via various pathways. Evidence also demonstrates that melatonin may attenuate edema and the ensuing tissue damage.[5]

The deep sleep stages of the sleep cycle also coincide with the release of growth hormone and other anabolic hormones important in the repair of muscle and other tissues from training.[6] More sleep cycles (that is, sleeping longer) means more of these anabolic hormones are released and more repair can occur.

Various aspects of the nervous system also recover during sleep.[7] This allows for enhanced learning and memory as well as reaction time and attentiveness.

In contrast, it has also been shown that sleep deprivation is associated with a host of negative health and performance problems including: obesity, diabetes, heart disease, stroke, increased blood pressure, the stress hormone cortisol, reduced immune function, depression, decreased motivation, overeating and poor nutritional choices, increased incidence of accidents, fatigue, increased perception of effort, and reduced performance.[8,9,10,11]

Not surprisingly, there is also evidence that insufficient sleep may increase the risk of overtraining syndrome in athletes.[12] On the cognitive side of the equation, which is arguably the primary area affected, chronic sleep deprivation results in decreased motivation, memory and learning; poor attention and concentration, all of which can have implications for learning and ingraining new running skills such as downhill and uphill techniques, improving running form, and knowing course details such as where and when to turn on the trail (I have had this happen to me a number of times, although I look at it as free miles from the Race Director!).[13]

Unfortunately for endurance athletes, we may be getting the short end of the sleeping stick, as the negative effects of sleep deprivation seem to be more pronounced in prolonged submaximal activities, which include distance running.[14]

To compound these problems, chronic sleep deprivation (three or more nights) has been shown to be cumulative, and is called *sleep debt*.[15] Sleep debt is analogous to a credit card where we borrow against the bank, but instead of paying it off right away, we get more and more in debt. Making the minimum payment of sleep on the weekend doesn't get us back to an even balance. Thankfully, there are a number of *foundational strategies to improve your sleep*.

First and foremost you need to know how much sleep you need. Research has shown there are large differences not only in how much sleep different people need, but also in how sleep deficit affects us.[16,17] Brain scanning studies indicate there is likely a genetic association responsible, at least in part, for these variances. On average it seems 7.5 to 9 hours is ideal. This range is based on sleep studies that have shown four to six sleep cycles of 90 minutes typically occur in people who wake well rested. There are five stages of sleep in a sleep cycle, with stages one to four known as non-REM (NREM) that represent progressively light to deep sleep, and the fifth stage being REM (rapid eye movement). For example, in stage one, you are easily woken, but someone in stages three or four is pretty hard to wake up, and when they are, they will be drowsy and "out of it." Stage four is also when growth hormone and other positive recovery processes are kicking in. REM is also not an optimal time to be woken and will result in feeling groggy. To find your personal sleep cycle duration, try using a sleep app. While not perfect (they are affected by someone else moving as they sleep) they are becoming more sophisticated and are relatively inexpensive compared to a sleep study at a medical facility.

Once you have an understanding of how much sleep you need, establish and stick to a regular schedule of going to bed and getting up that results in you feeling alert when you wake up. Go to bed and get up at the same time every day, including weekends.

Avoid using sleep medications if you can, unless prescribed by a physician. Some sleep aids can actually disrupt your sleep cycle, so even though you may be asleep for a longer period of time, the quality of sleep may be affected and you can still wake feeling tired.

Start winding down 20 minutes before getting into bed to allow your body and brain to start relaxing, which will allow for a more rapid and successful transition into stage one sleep. Have a warm shower, stretch, and avoid technology.

Avoid caffeine after 3 pm, even if you are a habitual user. Caffeine has a half-life (the time it takes for half the dose to be metabolized by enzymes in your liver) of about 4 hours. If you have a cup of coffee at 3 pm (100mg of caffeine), by 7 pm there will still be 50mg in your system. By 11 pm it will be cut in half again, down to 25mg. While those who regularly consume several caffeinated beverages a day might say they don't feel hyped up, caffeine is still active, even if at a lower sensitivity in these individuals.

For those who are experiencing sleep debt, in order to get back to normal sleep/wake cycles, experts have recommended that if you missed an average of 2 hours sleep a night during the week (e.g., 10 hours total), you need to repay that 10 hours and possibly another 4, and even more for some people.[18] One strategy to achieve this is to sleep an extra 2-3 hours per night on the weekend plus an extra hour a night during the subsequent week (because adding 2 hours extra during the work week is typically not possible for most people), and if needed, the remaining debt is repaid the following weekend. As you can see, getting back to normal sleep/wake levels can be demanding and prolonged.

Just like warming up and cooling down to reduce the risk of injury, prevention of sleep debt is better than the cure.

For those with *long-term sleep debt*, it can take many weeks or even months to get back to normal. An alternative is to have a sleep-time vacation! Get to bed on time and sleep in until you wake up on your own. My wife and I have four small children so that's not in the cards for either of us, but if you can, I hear it's amazing!

On the other end of the spectrum, getting an extra 2 hours sleep per night for several weeks has been found to increase athletic performance in a variety of sports including basketball and swimming.[19,20] So, sleep your way to improved race times!

A number of nutritional strategies have also been proposed to improve sleep and may also enhance recovery.[21] Diets high in protein or a high protein meal an hour or two before sleep may improve the quality of sleep, and also provide the necessary building blocks of muscle and protein to enhance repair from training. High glycemic index foods (those which raise blood glucose relative to white bread) such as white rice, bread, and potatoes, if consumed more than an hour before bed, may improve sleep. There is research which supports the notion that tryptophan, a naturally occurring amino acid which is converted to a compound called 5-HT and subsequently is converted to melatonin in the brain, makes you sleepy and enables better sleep.[22] Consuming approximately 300g of turkey or 200g of pumpkin seeds should provide about 1g of tryptophan which may be the minimum dose needed.

Lastly, what about having a nap? Does it help at all or is it just a short-term and short-lived fix?

Taking a 20-30 minute nap in the early afternoon can be a powerful tool to recover from a poor night of sleep.[23] Several studies have shown that such a nap can improve cognitive and sprint performance as well.[24] Only sleeping for 20-30 minutes means you stay in stage one and two of the sleep cycle without entering deep sleep, so it is easier to wake up and feel refreshed. For help in waking up, turn on the lights or step into the bright sunshine. Washing your face in cold water also helps wakefulness. An additional option is to consume a large caffeinated beverage before getting comfortable for your nap (which should be in a cool, dark, quiet place).[25] The caffeine and extra fluid making its way to your bladder will assist in helping you wake in a very alert state!

Sleep is a powerful and essential aspect of training, recovery, and physical and psychological health. Health is the cornerstone of a successful training program. If you're not healthy, you can't train effectively or consistently. You make time to train and eat right, and it's important that you also find time to get sufficient quality and quantity of sleep. Now, go catch some ZZZZZs!

Using Imagery to Run Your Best Marathon
Jay Johnson, MS

I strongly believe that runners need to use mental imagery to run to their potential on race day. Using imagery isn't complicated. Find a quiet space and imagine yourself going through the race. A quiet spot and 3-10 minutes is all it takes. I used imagery on and off during my collegiate career. There is no doubt that my best two races (a 14:20 5k on Friday night, and a 8:20 3k on Saturday afternoon, at the Big XII Indoor conference championships) were the result, in some part, of the mental imagery I used to prepare for the race. There were countless races where I didn't use imagery in the days leading up to the race, and, in retrospect, I think my performance suffered.

I recommend you start this process ten to fourteen days out from your marathon. Start with just 3 minutes a day, and as you get closer to the race, work your way up to roughly 10 minutes. As weird as it may sound, I find that sitting on the toilet in a bathroom is an ideal place to do this work. That said, don't use the port-a-potty as your quiet space on race day, keeping your fellow runners waiting to take care of their important business. You won't be very quiet, calm, or popular if you do.

The idea of mental imagery is to see yourself in the race: running the race and grooving the pace in the opening 20 miles, grabbing water and sports drinks with ease, taking a gel and having it go down easy, seeing runners pass you in the opening miles (runners who are going out too fast and will not doubt come back to you in the last 6.2 miles of the race), hearing the music at the start line, passing dozens of runners in the last 6.2 miles, and the crowd cheering at the first mile. You should be able to tune in to how your legs are going to feel, how your respiration will feel, and how your posture will feel. This all should feel good as you envision the first 20 miles.

In the first few imagery sessions you want to envision everything going well. Once you've made this positive picture in your head, it's time to envision things going wrong. See yourself going through a tough mile, or coming to a full stop at an aid station to get your water or sports drink. The key here is to envision something going wrong and then seeing yourself positively dealing with it.

Finally, what self-talk are you going to use in the final 6.2 miles of the marathon to help you grind out the last section? You can come up with your own version of Cindy Kuzma's, "You do hard things." The key is that you use imagery to hear yourself using positive self-talk to grind out the last 6.2 miles. Imagery is a powerful tool, so make sure to use it in the final ten days leading up to the marathon.

Caffeine Long Run
Carwyn Sharp, PhD

A quick nugget about refueling after your long run—you may think about adding a cup of coffee (or two or three) to your post-run meal. An interesting study showed that when subjects were glycogen depleted from cycling to fatigue (after doing exhausting intervals the night before and ingesting a low-carb meal) and then consumed a high carb meal (4 g/kg body weight) with a large dose of caffeine (8 mg/kg) during the next four hours of recovery, their muscle glycogen levels were on average 66% higher than those who only consumed the carbohydrates.[1]

A closer look at the specific details of this study however, could make you think twice. First, the dose of caffeine (8mg per kg body weight) for a 154 pound (70kg) individual is 560mg, which is equivalent to roughly 5.5 cups of coffee in four hours. Plus, they also consumed a LOT of carbohydrates (4g per kg body weight) – which for our 154 lbs person is 280g or approximately ten bananas. And lastly, if you have completed a ride or run to volitional fatigue, hopefully you don't need to replenish your fuel stores in the next few hours and you can have a rest.

The message here is that if you like a cup of coffee after your run (or ride) go ahead, it may improve your recovery. Science says, "You're welcome."

Delayed Onset Muscle
Soreness (DOMS)
Carwyn Sharp, PhD

Delayed Onset Muscle Soreness (DOMS) is mild to significant muscle pain, tenderness, inflammation, and swelling you experience after a particularly hard workout (greater intensity or duration), or a type of workout you are not used to. DOMS typically peaks 24-72 hours after the bout of exercise, depending on the extent or severity and how well-trained the athlete is, with evidence suggesting better trained athletes repair faster.[1] Peak DOMS coincides with peak muscle cell death about 48 hours after exercise.[2] Although this condition has been known for decades, the exact mechanisms that cause it are still not completely understood. What the scientific literature does indicate is that training which induces significant muscle micro-damage, and eccentric muscle contractions in particular, result in greater DOMS than concentric actions.[3,4] Eccentric contractions are when the muscles are being lengthened but the muscles are working hard to slow the lengthening. Running downhill is an example of this and causes certain muscles to work/contract to slow you down, but your momentum still carries you forward resulting in these muscles being lengthened as they are trying to contract and shorten.

No Pain No Gain, right? Not exactly. While DOMS is a sign that you have exerted yourself more than normal (which is a good thing, because we need to stress the body to adapt and improve), moderate and severe DOMS means you did much more than your body was prepared for. Also, the more severe your DOMS, the longer it lasts, and the more impact it has on your training. For example, the effects of DOMS on running has shown that even in well trained runners and triathletes, a bout of downhill running can result in significant DOMS and negative changes in range of motion, stride mechanics, running economy and an increased anaerobic energy production.[5] DOMS also causes a decrease in the ability to generate force with the affected muscle(s).[6] So, mild pain is okay and reflects a well-designed and appropriately progressing training program, but if you're debilitated after a workout, it's a sign you stepped things up too much and should dial it back.

We know that DOMS is, at least partly, the result of muscle damage from training (not lactic acid as some have proposed), however muscle damage has also been shown to be necessary to cause increases in muscle mass and strength, and may not cause pain or swelling. The extent of the damage appears to be important. File it under the Goldilocks principle: a little muscle damage forces the muscles to adapt and results in little pain (this is just right!), but more damage leads to DOMS and reflects overly aggressive training increases, and severe damage may lead to rhabdomyolysis, a potentially life threatening condition. Rhabdomyolysis is the rupture of significant amounts of muscle tissue, which causes the contents of these many muscle cells to leak into the blood. Some of these substances, such as myoglobin, cause kidney damage. This condition can be exacerbated by extremes in body temperature and severe dehydration.

As runners, we can't avoid eccentric muscle contractions, as there will always be some level of braking as our feet hit the ground (more so in novices than elites), and when running down hills. But the body is an amazing structure! Exposure to increasing doses of eccentric exercise, which may produce mild DOMS, will cause the body to adapt and be able to handle more eccentric exposure with less damage. So if you are new to hills, add them in so you have a progressive and sustainable overload of the muscles that they can handle. And remember, it is both the uphill and the downhill you are training to improve on!

What can you do about DOMS if you do step up training more than you should have, or the race course has many more hills than you thought? I experienced this on a purportedly "flat" Colorado half marathon, coming from coastal South Carolina and Texas. The hills caught me unprepared and I suffered a mild case of DOMS.

There are a number of strategies that can be employed to both avoid and recover from DOMS more quickly. Firstly, prevention is better than a cure. When running, shorten your stride and increase your cadence.[7] Overstriding increases the braking action when your foot hits the ground, which increases the amount of eccentric load with every stride.

Another preventative approach is to be better trained! There's evidence that better trained athletes need less protein to repair muscles than novices do.[8] As you continue through your marathon training program you will be better able to handle more difficult training that earlier in your training cycle might well have elicited a DOMS effect.

In conjunction with being better trained, another approach is to use the repeated bout effect. Simply put, an initial bout of eccentric exercise, such as downhill running or two to ten near-maximal eccentric lifts in the gym, will cause some DOMS (does not have to be significant), but will protect against DOMS in subsequent repeated bouts of DOMS-inducing exercise.[9,10] So yes, in this case, a little pain for a lot of pain avoidance! It doesn't mean you will never have DOMS again, but you may have increased your threshold.

Nutritionally, consuming a meal which contains carbohydrates and protein after endurance exercise enhances the recovery processes. One hundered grams of protein immediately after exercise significantly enhances recovery from measures of force and power in the 48 hours after a 30 minute downhill (-10°) run that induced significant DOMS.[11,12]

There is some evidence that indicates when caffeine is ingested in relatively high doses (5mg per kg body weight) 24 and 48 hours after DOMS-inducing eccentric exercise, it can significantly reduce pain and attenuate the force loss associated with DOMS.[13] It should be noted that the subjects were not habitual caffeine users, so whether this would work in individuals who regularly consume coffee or energy drinks is not known.

Interestingly, ice, cryotherapy, stretching, ultrasound, TENS (electrical stimulation therapy), and light exercise (such as a recovery run) do not seem to be effective at treating DOMS.[14] Ice may work as a mild analgesic (pain reducing agent) but only for a very short period of time, and it may in fact delay healing and recovery. While light exercise doesn't seem effective, the latest research is showing that moderate intensity aerobic exercise may be beneficial.[15]

Non-steroidal anti-inflammatories (NSAIDs) such as acetaminophen and ibuprofen may work in a dose-dependent manner as an analgesic, but recent studies have shown they seem to have no effect on inflammation after eccentric loading, and actually decrease protein synthesis and repair; they may result in a net effect of actually delaying healing.[16,17]

Debate continues on whether compression clothing worn during exercise has an effect on improving performance or enhancing recovery. There is growing evidence supporting the claims that graduated compression garments worn in the days after exercise inducing DOMS, can reduce soreness and weakness, and improve recovery.[18,19] Graduated compression is a key aspect as uniform compression does not seem effective.

DOMS is not an essential part of training, but it can serve as a sign that you are progressing too aggressively in your training program. If you do experience DOMS, there are various strategies, including nutritional strategies that you can use to enhance recovery. And yes, after recovery you will likely have adapted to be stronger, hopefully faster, and definitely more resilient to future DOMS!

Finding A Practitioner
Dr. Richard Hansen

Knowing whom to go to when an injury creeps up during training can be a confusing process. The assumption by many is that all practitioners, especially in the same profession, are alike. Selecting a provider would be much simpler if everyone's knowledge base, assessment of injuries (especially running-related), approach to care, and advice on how to appropriately return to normal training were the same. This unfortunately is not the case, and there are more bad providers than good. Keep this in mind: physician (medical doctor) advice doesn't always involve medications, physical therapy care doesn't always involve clam shell exercises and ultrasound, and chiropractic treatment doesn't always involve adjustments.

Bottom line when selecting a practitioner (regardless of specialty) for your injury: research what their experience is with running in general. This is key! It does make a difference when you're trying to explain to your doctor that your hamstring hurts after 10 miles of a 15 mile long run, but isn't noticeable during mile repeats. The practitioner's running-specific experience is just as important as the treatment techniques utilized and professional credentials.

As it relates to what type of practitioner to see, I'd start with a sports-specific chiropractor or physical therapist as your entry portal. Make sure the chiropractor is certified as CCSP (Certified Chiropractic Sports Practitioner) or DACBSP (Diploma of the American Chiropractic Board of Sports Physicians). Chiropractors and physical therapists can usually serve as your entry portal for more serious injuries and can help manage the more minor soft tissue injuries. Chiropractors also have the ability to order imaging and/or blood work if it is clinically indicated, which can help prevent delays in the diagnostic and rehab process.

Additionally, there are a few preferred soft tissue techniques that I feel are effective at treating most running injuries. Active Release Technique (A.R.T.), Graston Technique, dry needling, lymphatic massage, and joint mobilizations are the methods I tend to recommend, but the condition being treated and stage of severity play a big role in which technique is needed.

For minor muscle strains, nerve entrapments, and joint capsule dysfunctions, A.R.T. is the preferred method. It works by utilizing active patient motion of the involved area while the practitioner maintains tension along the tissue fibers in order to increase blood flow and improve flexibility.

For tendon and ligament injuries, Graston Technique and dry needling can be extremely helpful once the inflammatory phase of the injury has subsided. Graston Technique is an instrument-assisted form of soft tissue mobilization that targets adhesions and fascial restrictions associated with previous trauma or overuse. By stimulating fibroblastic proliferation, Graston Technique can help break down scar tissue and accelerate new tissue formation. Dry needling uses filiform or hypodermic needles to target overactive myofascial trigger points, eliciting a "local twitch response" within the tissue. This twitch response may signal the release of endogenous opiods helping to deactivate the trigger point and lower the pain threshold. Both Graston and dry needling techniques help to increase local blood supply to the treatment area, signaling a healing response in the hypoxic or damaged tissue.

Lymphatic massage is a form of gentle massage that targets the lymphatic system to improve fluid clearance and decrease pain associated with the inflammatory phase. This technique would be best utilized following a hard workout session, race, surgery, or acute injury to speed the clearance of waste products associated with acute skeletal muscle damage.

Joint mobilizations, especially low-grade amplitudes, can be utilized in most tissue recovery and injury rehab circumstances. This technique involves passively moving a joint through its range of motion to stimulate the mechanoreceptors of the joint, improving joint integrity and reducing pain.

Selecting the right practitioner with experience treating running injuries is crucial to ensuring an accurate diagnosis of your injury and preventing delays in the recovery process. There are many different technique systems available, but understanding the purpose behind each one and why it is beneficial for your specific situation is crucial to improving treatment outcomes.

Practice Makes Perfect (or at
least better prepared)
Cindy Kuzma, Freelance Writer
Contributing Editor to
Runner's World

I train for the Boston Marathon with a group based in Chicago—we do long runs on the Lakefront Trail or out in a hilly suburb called South Barrington, about an hour away from the city. Whichever route we're taking that day, we start at 8 a.m., January through April.

While I have my evening-before and morning-of routines down pat for these training runs, all that goes out the window on race day. Because it's a point-to-point course, we stay in a hotel in Boston and take a bus out to the starting line in Hopkinton, leaving at 6 a.m. sharp. We're among the first to reach the Athlete's Village and are fortunate enough to be able to stay cozy and shielded from the elements on our chartered buses until we head to the starting line. But depending on your wave—I'm usually in the second one—that might not be until 10 a.m., 11 a.m., or even later.

Each year I've struggled with this shift, unsure of what to eat and when, how to occupy my brain while waiting, the proper balance of conserving energy by relaxing on the bus and loosening up my legs by walking around a bit. My fourth year of running Boston, in 2015, I knew I was in shape to run my best time yet. So I decided to get a little more serious about fine-tuning my morning.

I chose one of my long runs to do on my own and treated it as a dress rehearsal for the whole event. I paid close attention to what I ate and when the night before, having dinner earlier than I would on a normal day (since our group meal in Boston starts at 5 p.m.). I got up around 5, got dressed, and carried breakfast, snacks, and coffee to my husband's recliner. There I sat for the approximately 45 minutes it takes to drive the length of the course backward. I allowed myself to get up to use the bathroom—we have one on the bus, after all—but otherwise I read magazines or snoozed in a similar position to a bus seat.

Once I'd "arrived," I took a few quick walks outside, as we often do on race morning (besides using the porta-potties—that bus bathroom gets less fresh after carting a load of runners—we have to snap the requisite photo next to the "It All Starts Here" sign in Hopkinton). But each time, I'd return to the chair-bus for a snack or a swig of Gatorade. Shortly before the time I'd be starting my wave, I headed outside and walked—rather than ran—to the lakefront (I'm lucky enough to live a little less than a mile away from the trail—just about perfect, since it's about three-quarters of a mile's hike from the Athlete's Village to the starting line).

When race day arrived a few weeks later, I felt much more confident in my routine—and did, indeed, beat my best Boston time by about a minute. Of course, I did a lot of hard training and other mental preparation work to achieve this goal! But I definitely believe the dry run went a long way toward helping me feel relaxed and *in-the-groove* on race morning. After all, I'd grooved it all before, just a few weeks prior.

> The Last 6.2 Miles
> of a Marathon
> Amy Feit, Working Mom
> Marathon PR of 2:58:13

Prior to working with Jay, my approach to the last 6.2 miles of a marathon was the try-to-hold-on-for-dear-life method. As you can imagine, this never worked out well. I spent so much energy planning every detail of the opening miles of the marathon—every mile had a specific pace in mind. With a pace band strapped to my wrist, I would set out for my race and almost always nail the first 20 miles. I was going to do whatever was needed to hit those paces. However, after hitting 20 mile, the anticipation would begin. I would just wait for the moment where I would begin to fall apart; and I inevitably fell apart, every single time. The breakdown came in many forms—calf cramping, heavy legs, and most of all, mentally not having the fortitude to continue at the pace of the first 20 miles.

Jay's *groove and grind* method has proven over and over to be a much better way to attack the marathon distance. Jay has me *groove* for the first 20 miles. The most challenging portion of the race is being patient and restraining myself from going faster than I should the first 20 miles. After months of hard training and going into the race rested and with fresh legs, it is very difficult to not push the pace in the opening half of the race. I almost always feel like I could be running faster in the first half of the race and it is very hard to fight the urge to go faster. I spend many of the first 20 miles telling myself to relax and to not let things get out of hand. Not every mile feels good. There is of course, the inevitable mile 9, or 16, or whatever the mile might be, that feels overly hard. I tell myself to push through and it will pass; and it always does.

Once I hit the 20-mile mark, it's game on! This is the point where I really feel like I get to race. The first 20 miles I spend restraining myself and now it is time to let 'er buck. It is at mile 20 when I open up that the really hard work begins. The game plan is to break down the last 6.2 miles into chunks. Three miles, 2 miles, and then 1.2 miles. The first 3 miles I am telling myself, "you can totally hold this pace for another 3 miles." After being patient the first 20 miles, 3 more miles at the same pace is a very doable task. I remind myself throughout these 3 miles that I am going to have to push a bit harder in order to maintain pace.

Once I get to mile 23, I start the game over and count down 2 more miles. This is probably the hardest part of the last 6.2 of a marathon. However, by breaking it down into a 2-mile segment, I am able to just focus on the mile I am currently running. In the first mile I am telling myself to just keep pushing and then I'll soon only have one more mile before I can say I'm on the last mile. It is in these 2 miles that I spend a lot of mental energy trying to stay on task. At this point I feel as though I am running as fast and as hard as I can. To get through these 2 miles I spend a lot of time focusing on people and landmarks ahead of me. "Reel in the guy in the red hat," "Make it past that bridge," "Don't take your eyes off the gal in the pink compression socks until you pass her,"—these are all tactics I use.

The biggest motivator at this point in the race is that I am now passing a lot of runners. By being patient and smart in the first 20 miles, seeing runners that passed me come back into view is fuel for the fire in the late miles.

By mile 25, I do somewhat deploy the hold-on-for-dear-life method. It's a whole different story when I am trying to do it for 1.2 miles versus 6.2 miles. In the last mile it does take every ounce of strength I have left to keep going at the pace I have been carrying on at for the previous 25 miles. I am solely focused on the finish line during the last mile and it is such a glorious and fulfilling moment to cross that finish line having run the last 6.2 miles intelligently and strong!

The Science of
Optimizing Fueling During
the Marathon
Trent Stellingwerff, PhD

Most marathoners will expend over 2,500 to 3,000 kcals of energy to complete a marathon. Given the reality that most athletes only have ~2,000 kcals of muscle glycogen, maximizing the amount of energy and carbohydrate (CHO) they can deliver to their muscles during the race is fundamental. Furthermore, contrary to popular belief, the few studies that have directly measured substrate oxidation over prolonged intense endurance exercise (~2 to 5h) in well-trained, non-fat adapted subjects, have shown these exercise durations to be very CHO dominant (>70% of total energy expenditure (EE) when consuming CHO.[1] This short review will examine both the laboratory and field research, and outline contemporary recommendations on maximizing CHO intake and utilization (oxidation) during prolonged endurance sports, such as marathons.

Proposed Mechanism For Performance Enhancement

The exact mechanism(s) of fatigue, and thus what limits performance, are multi-factorial in nature. Furthermore, the impact that carbohydrate (CHO) supplementation can have on metabolism and performance depends on the length and intensity of the exercise as well as the CHO dose (intake rate) and type of carbohydrate. Thus, the mechanisms and regulation involved with fuel metabolism and energy production during exercise are very complex. However, there have been two major mechanisms that have emerged to primarily explain why CHO supplementation improves performance, and these are: 1) a stimulation of the central nervous system (CNS) by CHO when muscle and liver glycogen energy stores are not limiting via oral exposure and 2) direct contribution of CHO energy and CHO oxidation during situations of low-glycogen availability (e.g., late during prolonged exercise). The former generally occurs during exercise durations of less than 1 hour, while the latter generally occurs during exercise situations of greater than 2h, and would certainly be the major mechanism responsible for any performance benefits during a marathon race.

Although there are many factors to prolonged endurance exercise fatigue (>2h), beyond just fuel provision to the muscle, the primary mechanism for this improved performance has been an enhanced maintenance of plasma glucose (prevention of hypoglycemia), which results in increased CHO oxidation (utilization) by the muscles during exercise. However, the question remains: can more carbohydrate, and hence greater CHO oxidation, further improve performance? It appears that the rate-limiting step to CHO oxidation is at the level of the gastro-intestinal (GI) tract due to the intestinal CHO transport mechanisms; specifically the activity of the SGLT 1 transporter for glucose and the GLUT-5 transporter for fructose.[2] It is thought that having a high uptake and oxidation efficiency of supplemented CHO beverages should reduce the accumulation of CHO in the gastro-intestinal (GI) tract and in turn reduce the potential for GI distress during exercise. This point is not trivial, as even minor GI distress is associated with negative endurance performance outcomes.

Laboratory Evidence For CHO Intake To Improve Endurance Performance

Several recent laboratory studies evaluated the combined ingestion of a sports drink containing glucose + fructose or maltodextrin + fructose in a 2:1 ratio (multi-transportable CHOs) and at an ingestion rate of ~1.8 g/ min on oxidation rate of exogenous CHO (for review see: [2]). This pattern of multi-transportable CHO ingestion resulted in ~20 to 50% higher CHO oxidation compared with the ingestion of a drink containing an isocaloric amount of glucose or maltodextrin only. In a recent systematic review, 82% of investigations (n=50 studies) demonstrated statistically greater endurance performance or capacity with carbohydrate (CHO) intake when compared with water alone.[3] Additionally, nearly every single study demonstrates a performance benefit of CHO intake, with the effect on performance ever increasing with prolonged exercise time (r=0.356; p<0.01). Further, multi-transportable CHOs have an even greater impact on performance when exercise is longer than 2h ($9.6 \pm 4.8\%$ increase in performance), compared to only $4.3 \pm 2.7\%$ increase with single-source CHOs (e.g., glucose alone).

Practical Field Recommendations

Indirect correlative data also supports the notion that the more CHO an athlete can tolerate, the better endurance performance will be during prolonged exercise.[4] Furthermore, we have previously found a highly significant correlation between endurance athletes who have a history of GI problems during exercise and measured GI problems during competition, with about 15 to 20% of endurance athletes having a chronic history of GI problems.[4]

Taken together, it appears that there is a large diversity of CHO oxidation and GI responses, and that each endurance athlete will have a unique "sweet spot" where the athlete is able to absorb and oxidize a maximum amount of CHO/fluids to improve endurance performance versus too much fluids and CHO, which will cause GI distress and decrease performance. This individual variability is reflected in a recently-published elite-marathon nutrition and training case study, showing a self-selected range from 49 to 77g CHO/hr in 3 elite marathoners during sub 2:12 marathon efforts.[5]

This wide range of actual and recommended CHO intake depends on the CHO type, the individual, and the mode and intensity of the exercise intervention, as outlined in the figure below, and probably best reflects the wide ranges actually found, and well-tolerated, in the field with athletes.[4,5] Therefore, it is imperative that athletes practice and develop an individualized fueling and hydration plan prior to any competition, which can be tracked and monitored into a tracking sheet (Table 1).

Sweat, Fluid, And Carbohydrate Worksheet

Date			
Temp			
Humidity			
Pre-Run (Weight kg)			
Post-Run (Weight kg)			
Amount of Fluids Ingested (L)			
Total Amount of CHOs consumed (grams)			
Time Run (hrs or fraction of hrs)			
Fluid Intake Rate (L/hr)			
CHO Intake Rate (CHO/hr)			
Sweat Rate (L/hr)			
% Body Weight Loss			
Comments (feelings, GI effects, etc.)			

Table 1. Example of an individualized fueling and hydration tracking sheet. Track information into spreadsheet/work tool to find out what your individual sweat rate and fueling intake abilities are. Note: CHO = Carbohydrate (in grams)

Practical fueling and hydration recommendations during exercise include:
- In every session longer than ~75min, track sweat rate in different weather conditions, especially in targeted race weather conditions— track information into worksheet.
- Practice fueling and hydration in every long run. Practice with different amounts of fluids and fuels, mimicking the timing of intake in your race (~15 to 20min)—track information into worksheet. Ideally practice

under race pace intensities! Especially focus on practicing your race-day fueling protocol at least 8 to 10 weeks prior to your target marathon.

- Aim for at least 40g of carbs/h and >500ml/h water to start, but try and really "test" your GI and see what you can handle. The more you can adapt and handle taking in carbohydrate, the more fuel you will have at the end of the race. Ideally, you can adapt to hit >60g CHO/h or more when running and >90g CHO/h cycling.

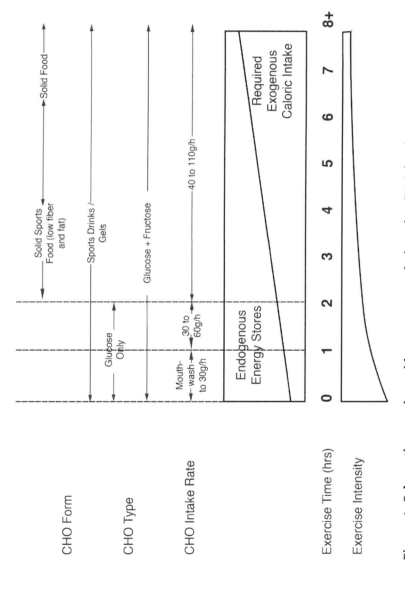

Figure 1. Schematic overview of key recommendations for CHO intake rate, CHO type and form over varying exercise durations and intensities.

The Science of
Heat and Hydration
Trent Stellingwerff, PhD

As a result of the inefficiency of metabolic transfer, >75% of the energy that is generated by skeletal muscle during exercise is liberated as heat, with only ~25% going to power or speed generation. During exercise, several powerful physiological mechanisms of heat loss are activated to prevent an excessive rise in body core temperature. However, exercising in the heat presents various challenges as metabolic heat from the body is coupled with environmental heat, inducing a greater physiological strain than would occur in temperate conditions. Heat generated by contracting muscles during exercise increases body core temperature, which in turn causes blood flow to be redirected to the skin for peripheral blood vessel dilation and sweating.[1] As a result, the body's central metabolic demand competes with the heat loss requirements of the skin, resulting in an early onset of cardiovascular strain that can adversely impact athletic performance. A cardiovascular inefficiency results in attempt to maintain this central blood volume and is characterized by a decrease in stroke volume and cardiac output due to a loss of plasma water in the blood. Sweat rate increases in a feed-forward mechanism in hot and humid environments in response to a depleted blood volume.[1] This in turn results in a greater loss of plasma water in the blood, which induces stress on whole-body water stores.[2] It is common for athletes engaging in high intensity exercise in hyper-thermic conditions to have sweat rates of 1.0-2.5L/hour and sweat rates of >2.5L/hour are not uncommon in high ambient temperatures or in large athletes.[2]

Optimal Marathon Weather Conditions And Impact Of Heat On Performance

In a series of studies, Ely et al. examined the ideal weather conditions for optimal marathon performance.[3] The common factor among fast marathon performances has been low temperature (~11-13°C/52-55°F, for males and 12-14°C/54-57°F for females), while the presence of cloud cover or low solar load does not increase the likelihood of running a fast marathon. In further mathematical modeling, they showed that a 25°C/77°F marathon day would, on average, decrease marathon performance by ~3% in a 2:10 marathoner, and a large 12% reduction in performance in a 3hr marathoner. In other words, the negative impact of heat can be large in marathon performance.

Measuring Sweat Rates And Losses During Training

Below are some practical recommendations on how you can measure your own sweat rates during training, based on the principle that 1kg = 1L of sweat. The calculation of sweat rate quantifies the amount of fluids lost, providing more tangible guidelines for fluid replacement. The following is a simple step-by-step breakdown of sweat rate calculation. Since it takes 30-40 minutes to fully "turn on" sweating, this calculation can underestimate sweat rates when used for exercise periods of short duration.

1. Equipment required: weigh scale (accurate to 0.1kg), stopwatch, and a pre-measured water bottle in milliliters (ml).
2. Measure body weight to the nearest 0.1kg prior to exercise.
3. Measure volume of fluids to be ingested during exercise (in ml) and place in water bottle.
4. Start stopwatch when exercise begins, drink fluid as normal, record volume of fluid left at end of session.
5. Stop stopwatch when exercise ends, record time.
6. Take post-exercise body weight (make sure you are dry and that all wet clothing has been removed).
7. Measure out any remaining fluids from water bottle, record leftover measurement (in ml).

Calculation	Sample Calculation
Deficit = (pre weight – post weight) x 1000	Pre weight: 51.0 kg
Pre weight: _____ (kg)	Post weight: 50.0 kg
Post weight: _____ (kg)	**Deficit** = (51.0 kg – 50.0 kg) x 1000
Deficity: _____ (kg) x 1000	= 1.0 kg x 1000
	= 1000 ml
% Body Mass Lost = (deficit / 10) / pre weight	**% Body Mass lost** = (1000 / 10) / 51.0
	= 1.96% body weight
Fluid Intake = (pre fluids – post fluids)	Pre fluids: 1000 ml
Pre Fluids: _____ (ml)	Post fluids: 250 ml
Post Fluids: _____ (ml)	**Fluid Intake** = (1000 ml – 250 ml)
	= 750 ml
Sweat Loss = deficit (ml) + fluid intake (ml)	**Sweat Loss** = 1000 ml + 750 ml
	= 1750 ml or 1.75 L
Time = practice duration or exercise time	**Time** = 45 minutes
= # of minutes / 60 minutes (per hour)	= 45 minutes / 60 minutes (per hour)
	= 0.75 hours
Sweat rate = sweat loss / time	**Sweat rate** = 1.75 L / 0.75 hours
	= 2.33 L / hour

Table 2. Example of sweat rate calculations

Practical Hydration Strategies

- Develop individualized re-hydration plans well in advance. Each athlete may respond to the heat and humidity in unique ways. Before competitions in the heat, determine during training how much each athlete needs to drink before, during, and after exercise in order to avoid dehydration (practice this at home in different weather conditions by looking at pre- to post-training body weight, see below).

- Advise the athletes to drink beyond the sensation of thirst, especially during the initial acclimatization to heat and humidity.

- Begin all training and competition well hydrated. If possible drink throughout, but in small amounts to avoid sensation of 'bloating'.

- Accurate hydration status can be monitored with Urine Specific Gravity strips or Urine Osmolarity assay. Your team physiologist and/or nutritionist should be able to provide further information on these testing protocols.

- As you will be in a new environment, with not only different temperatures, but also food choices, it is recommended to regularly monitor morning weight prior to championships. Large decreases or gains should be discussed with the medical staff who can offer advice.

- Measure body weight before and after training to determine water loss and % body weight loss. It is normal for exercise to induce more than ~2 to 3% body weight loss. More than 4% means you did not drink enough, less than 2% means you drank too much! [1Kg weight loss = 1 Liter water loss]; rehydrate with 1.5 L.

- Hydration supplements (which may contain carbohydrates, electrolytes, etc.) should be tested well in advance and in consultation with your sports nutritionist. Caution: If re-hydration is the goal, drinks with high sugar content will slow down the rate of water absorption from the stomach. If re-hydrating with an energy drink, the solution should contain ~2-3% carbohydrate.

- Athletes should be aware of their urine color when well hydrated. If the color is 4 or above (see *SimpleMarathonTraining.com*), they are already dehydrated enough to negatively impact performance. Note that urine color is affected by vitamin supplements.

- Athletes can over-hydrate and flush out electrolytes. Urine should be pale yellow, not clear! If you are waking during the night to urinate more than two times, you are probably over-hydrated.

To see the urine color test table go to *SimpleMarathonTraining.com*.

The Science of Heat Acclimation
Trent Stellingwerff, PhD

As outlined in the previous article on heat and hydration, there can be a large negative performance effect of both heat and dehydration on endurance performance. However, beyond attempts at hydrating, for both physiological and psychological benefits during exercise, recent research has also shown large positive performance benefits of short-term (5 to 10 days) heat acclimation protocols on performance outcomes—both racing in the heat and on cool and mild race days. This short review will look at the mechanisms of heat acclimation, including some practical protocols, to best deal with heat on race day.

Mechanisms Of Heat Acclimation To Improve Heat Tolerance And Performance

Elevated core temperatures initiate several mechanisms designed to dissipate heat, including sweating to cool skin via evaporation and dilation of peripheral skin blood vessels, which shunt heated blood from the core to the skin for cooling. Both of these mechanisms rely on the maintenance of blood volume (BV). Maintaining BV becomes very difficult in the heat because of the additive effects of heat generated from exercise combined with heat from the environment.[1] As a result, sweat rate increases in a feed-forward mechanism, resulting in a potentially greater loss of body fluids, which further compromises BV. If too much fluid is lost due to high sweat rates, cooling supersedes exercise, decreasing work rate, with the potential for complete shut-down (e.g., heat stroke).

Heat acclimation is a process which elicits physiological changes allowing an individual to deal with heat stress more effectively. Heat acclimation usually involves exercise in significant heat (>30°C/86°F with >50% humidity for 5 to 7 consecutive days) to elicit the optimal adaptations. One of the biggest adaptations is an increase in BV, specifically the plasma volume (PV), with some studies showing a ~5 to 7% increase in PV.[2,3,4] There are generally three benefits of increasing the circulating PV: 1) less competition between cooling and fueling exercising muscles, 2) more fluids available for sweating resulting in enhanced cooling capabilities, and 3) better maintenance and/or increase of cardiac output, and accordingly, ability to achieve greater VO²max values at maximal exercise, which have shown benefits in both warm and cool conditions (especially important to high intensity sports).[3]

Beyond changes in PV, there are a host of other adaptations that occur during heat acclimation, usually grouped as shorter-term adaptations (<5 days of heat acclimation), and longer-term adaptations (10-14 days of heat exposure).[5] Short-term adaptations include: an increase in PV and thermal comfort/perception, decreases in core and skin temperature, and large decreases in HR at sub-maximal exercise intensities. Longer-term adaptations include: increases in total sweat rates (once PV has increased), which eventually translates into 5 to 15% increase in performance capacity in the heat.[5]

Practical Heat Tolerance Strategies
- Modify the normal warm-up period (e.g., shorten time and reduce intensity) so that athletes do not overheat prior to important training or competition days.
- Establish pre-and post-cooling strategies, which can include ice baths, or even 'ice/cold water' towels in a hand-cooler that can be transported to the track, or even for field events, onto the field of play. Seek expert advice from your sport physiologist regarding performance and recovery cooling strategies.
- Minimize "accumulative heat load" between training sessions by avoiding mid-day socializing, sightseeing, shopping in the sun and heat, etc.
- Choose light and breathable clothing. Dark-colored clothing will absorb more radiant heat and thus add to the heat load. Ensure clothing does not restrict evaporation of sweat.
- Athletes, coaches, and team managers should be aware of the symptoms related to heat illness: headache, nausea, dizziness, excessive sweat,

loss of coordination. Seek medical advice for any of these symptoms. Be aware that some common headache medications are vasoconstrictors and may reduce the body's ability to dissipate heat.

- Keep cool at night to ensure good sleep. Quality sleep is critical for recovery and regeneration. Cool showers and ice-tubs can assist in this!

Practical Heat Acclimation Protocol

- A minimum of 7-14 days of heat acclimatization is required for complete adaptation. Allowing sweat rates to increase, decreasing the amount of sodium lost in sweat, resting and exercising heart rates to return to normal, and resting body temperature to return to normal. During the initial days of training in hot weather, the volume, intensity, and duration should be reduced to help the athlete adapt to the added heat stress.

- If coming from a cool environment, simulated heat exposure (such as use of a steam room) during the few weeks prior to departure will advance the rate of acclimatization. There are two primary approaches that have shown positive heat acclimation:

  - Sauna studies: 12 sauna visits over a ~3 week period, at ~90°C/194°F sauna for 30 min per visit.

  - Low-intensity exercise: 5 to 10 low-grade exercise exposures (>75min easy/moderate run) over ~5 to 10 days at ~30-35°C/86-95°F at >~50% humidity. Increase intensity as it gets easier. This can easily be done by setting up a treadmill in a small room with a heater, while possibly wearing layers of clothing.

- This is an acute intervention that would be implemented in the immediate weeks prior to a targeted competition. It is not necessary to implement this when already training in hot and humid conditions. This is only needed when training conditions are cool to temperate (<25°C/77°F and ~50% humidity).

- A recent study has shown that protein supplementation can help support the increase in blood plasma volume and accelerate adaptation to the heat.[6] Therefore, immediately post heat acclimation run or sauna, consume ~0.3g protein (e.g., whey) per kg BW (~20g of protein).

Pool Walking
Dr. Richard Hansen

Standing on the starting line of any race, it's natural for runners to run down the checklist of, "How does my body feel, and will it do what I hope it can today?" Soreness is a natural and common occurrence with any training plan. It's the response of our bodies trying to adapt to a new stimulus. When soreness lingers or the sensation turns to pain, it can inevitably raise concerns that the goal on race day is slip sliding away.

Reduce this fear by utilizing one of the easiest and most efficient recovery tools: pool walking. A pressure gradient is created the deeper your tissue is below the surface, which helps to prevent pooling of inflammation and move lymphatic fluid. For example, if you are standing at a depth of 4.5 feet of water, you are creating a pressure gradient equivalent to 77 mmHg at your calf (approximately 3.5 feet below the surface). This is over 2x greater than standard graduated athletic compression socks or sleeves (which are usually around 22-32 mmHg). Now, add walking to this equation and you create a joint pumping mechanism called imbibition to help mobilize the joint and further aid circulatory flow.

Additionally, pool walking can provide a valuable benefit in assisting muscle repair following a hard workout. Resting blood flow response in muscles has been shown to increase from 1.8ml/min/100g of tissue *not in water* compared to 4.1ml/min/100g *in water*. This means that pool walking is 225% more efficient at assisting oxygen supply to muscle tissue than walking on dry land, which is a crucial process for tissue repair.

Aqua therapy is also a commonly used rehabilitation practice for spinal cord injury patients due to a reduction in pain threshold noted when irritated tissue is submerged. Following intense bouts of running exercise, over-stimulus of the nervous system is a common occurrence. Having the ability to calm down the nervous system following intense or prolonged workouts can improve pain perception and decrease tissue sensitivity.

The challenge is finding time to get to the pool or finding access to a pool in your area. Try to pair pool walking days with workout days requiring gym equipment (e.g., squat racks, elliptical machines, free weights, etc.). This way the trip to the gym can be multi-faceted, saving you time and money. Keep yourself healthier by utilizing one of the most efficient and effective recovery tools available – the pool!

Cardiac Drift
Jay Johnson, MS

Cardiac drift is important for runners to understand, especially when running in heat and/or humidity. It's a very simple principle. When an athlete is running at the same effort (e.g., the same workout output) for 10 minutes or more and their heart rate "drifts" upward, the athlete is experiencing cardiac drift.

For the runner who can run by feel, an example may be an easy Wednesday run of 70 minutes. The runner is confident she is running a consistent effort is the same throughout the run, yet if she were wearing a heart rate monitor she would see her heart rate steadily increase over the course of the run. Why does this tend to happen when you run on a hot and/or humid day?

The body needs to cool itself, which means that you need to sweat to cool to maintain a stable core temperature. You are going to convert some of your blood plasma into sweat, which means that unless you bring in more liquids, the blood your heart is pumping is going to become more and more viscous compared to normal blood. The heart has to pump more rapidly as the viscosity of the blood rises, thus the correlation between sweating more and an increase in heart rate.

Because you won't be training with a heart rate monitor in the SMT system, you probably won't even notice this phenomenon occurring. That said, hydration is key to running your best on hot and/or humid days. For more information on the topic of hydration, please read Dr. Trent Stellingwerff's Geek Out on The Science of Heat and Hydration on page 202.

Growth Mindset
Travis Macy
Ultra Endurance Racer
Auhtor of *The Ultra Mindset*

Years of experience as an athlete, teacher, and coach have taught me that a subtle distinction in mindset can lead to a significant difference in improved performance, health, and enjoyment in running.

I learned about growth mindset vs. fixed mindset when I read Carol Dweck's excellent text, *Mindset*. The book made such an impact that I started teaching about it every week in my high school English classes. I subsequently wrote about the growth mindset as related to endurance training/racing and life in general in *The Ultra Mindset: An Endurance Champion's 8 Core Principles for Success in Business, Sports, and Life*.

Someone with a growth mindset, simply put, focuses on *getting better*; one who adopts the opposite—the fixed mindset—focuses on *being good*. The difference is subtle, yet revolutionary.

After a D on a test, a growth mindset student recognizes that he is not quite where he wants to be in, say, math, and then he works harder. The fixed mindset student comes to a different conclusion: "I struggle at math, so I shouldn't even try."

A corporate professional in the fixed mindset sees her colleague recognized for excellent sales and then gets jealous and competitive, reacting with gossip, an extra drink, and web searching for a new job. The mutual colleague with a growth mindset congratulates the awardee and asks her how he can work more skillfully to boost his own numbers.

Start looking for growth vs. fixed mindsets, and you'll see them just about everywhere in life. You'll also see them on the roads, trails, and track as you prepare for your marathon. Early in my running career, I made some poor choices based on a fixed mindset:

- Using training runs—rather than races—as a proving ground
- Running too hard on recovery days
- Doing too many runs with guys who were faster than me, which was particularly degrading on recovery days
- Paying more attention to weekly mileage and pace (and how they

211

looked to teammates/coaches/social media) than to how I actually felt and how I was progressing

Accordingly, I found myself overtrained, frustrated, and experiencing a plateau in performance. Shifting to a growth mindset made a big difference for me.

Like all runners, I am still a work in progress. That said, a growth mindset that has come with maturity has engendered some better decisions:

- Racing in the races and training in the training
- Listening to my body, resting when I need rest
- Staying away from training that leads to injury and burnout
- Doing most of my training according to time and perceived exertion and/or heart rate, rather than by pace and mileage (this decision is also a factor of training at high altitude on hilly, technical trails)
- Focusing on a self-concept that is not heavily based on proving my worth through running performances

Keep this in mind: the purpose of training is to get better. This seems obvious, but if you slip into a fixed mindset, you'll soon be using workouts to prove yourself instead of to progress gradually. If you explore running websites and articles with a fixed mindset, you'll probably start feeling bad about yourself because you're not as fast, or don't run as many miles, or have less experience.

Race with a purely fixed mindset and you'll be ruled by fear (of not making your time, of not finishing, of getting beat by your training partner, of "failing" in some other way). Race in a growth mindset and you'll have fun, get faster, enjoy the journey, and participate in running in a sustainable and life-changing manner. It's all about getting better, folks. Go get 'em with the growth mindset!

GEEK OUT
CONTRIBUTORS

Amy Feit

Amy lives and trains in the extreme and often harsh weather conditions of southwest Minnesota. She is lucky enough to have her passion for running supported by the ones she loves the most: her two daughters, Brooke and Regan, along with her husband Kyle. A recent new addition to her training support network is her running buddy for most easy days—an English Setter puppy named Wallace. Balancing family, marathon training, and a full-time career with a software company is a challenge made easier by being fortunate enough to work with wonderful people that follow and cheer her on through her racing endeavors.

Alia Gray

Alia Gray is a professional distance runner who trains in Boulder, Colorado with the Roots Running Project. Joe Vigil writes her training from afar. She has run 15:35 for the 5k, 31:59 for the 10k, 1:12:48 for the half marathon, and 2:35:47 for the marathon. She finished in 10th place at the 2016 US Olympic marathon trials with one of the few PRs set on a hot day. She also doubles as a freelance copywriter. She is an avid baker, coffee drinker, and foodie, and she loves checking out a good concert in her free time.

Dr. Richard Hansen, DC, DACBSP, CSCS

Dr. Richard Hansen is a chiropractor in Boulder, Colorado with a specialty in sports medicine. He holds the distinction of Sports Physician Diplomate (DACBSP), the highest credentialing awarded to sports chiropractors, and is a certified strength and conditioning specialist (CSCS). He routinely lectures on proper distance running training, sports injury management, and implementation of strength and conditioning for runners. He has had the opportunity to work with over 20 Olympians and has been a medical provider at the USATF Outdoor Championships, as both personal medical and on the USATF staff. Dr. Hansen is a former collegiate distance runner for UC San Diego and has coached every level of distance runner from youth to adult level athletes. He currently coaches a professional running group called Roots Running Project and owns a private sports medicine practice in Boulder, Colorado called High Altitude Spine and Sport.

Cindy Kuzma

Cindy Kuzma is a freelance health and fitness writer and a contributing editor at Runner's World magazine. She grew up in Texas and moved to Chicago to earn her master's in journalism at Northwestern University. Once she saw the lakefront running trail, she decided to stay. She's since finished 15 marathons (including four trips to Boston) and has also written for Men's Health, SELF, Prevention, Women's Health, and many other publications. You can read her work at *www.cindykuzma.com*.

Travis Macy

Finisher of over 120 ultra endurance events in 17 countries, Travis Macy is a speaker, author, coach, and professional endurance athlete. He is the author of *The Ultra Mindset: An Endurance Champion's 8 Core Principles for Success in Business, Sports, and Life*. Travis holds the record for the Leadman epic endurance event consisting of a trail running marathon, 50-mile mountain bike race, the Leadville 100 Mountain Bike Race, 10k road run, and the Leadville 100 Run, all above 10,200 feet of elevation in the Colorado Rockies.

Doug Petrick

Doug Petrick is a high school Physics teacher and coach at Upper St. Clair High School in Pittsburgh, Pennsylvania. He implements Coach Jay's philosophy into training his athletes year round for the cross country, indoor track and field, and spring track and field teams. An avid runner, Doug follows sound training principles to keep balance in his life as a teacher, coach, father of three, and husband. He values growth and development in all areas of his life and considers himself blessed to make a living doing what he loves. Doug continues to evolve as a coach and chase personal records through his own running.

Carwyn Sharp PhD, CSCS*D, USATF

Dr. Carwyn Sharp is a recognized expert in endurance sports who has authored and co-authored numerous book chapters, scientific articles, abstracts, presented at international and national conferences and clinics, and has been interviewed by publications such as Runner's World, Men's Fitness, Muscle & Fitness, MSN Healthy Living, and The New York Times.

Dr. Sharp is an exercise scientist with degrees in exercise physiology (BS, MS) and nutrition (PhD) who applies this knowledge as a coach (certified strength and conditioning specialist and USA Track and Field) and to himself (personal best marathon of 2:46).

Dr. Sharp is currently the Chief Science Officer for the National Strength & Conditioning Association, and previously worked at NASA's Johnson Space Center as the project scientist for Exercise Countermeasures, and also as an assistant professor researching the roles of high intensity training and nutrition on endurance performance and recovery.

Most importantly, he is a loving and devoted husband (I love you Sherri!) and father to four children, aged 1 to 10 years (Lyla, Christian, Ansley, and Connor—you are truly amazing and a blessing that I hold dear every day. Love you all heaps!).

Trent Stellingwerff PhD

Dr Trent Stellingwerff is a former Div. I NCAA runner (Cornell University), and currently serves as the director of innovation & research and lead of performance services at the Canadian Sport Institute Pacific (Victoria, Canada). In this role, he directs 15 different major research projects across different sport performance discipline areas, with six PhD to master's students involved. His primary sport and research focuses are via his physiology and nutrition expertise primarily to Canada's national Olympic rowing and track and field teams, with consulting roles to Cycling Canada and Triathlon Canada. Prior to this, Trent was a senior scientist in performance nutrition for PowerBar at the Nestle Research Center (Lausanne, Switzerland). Trent has more than sixty-five peer-reviewed scientific publications in major scientific and medical journals in the areas of exercise physiology, skeletal muscle metabolism, and performance nutrition and supplementation. He has co-authored five book chapters focusing on the role that nutrition can play in supporting elite athlete performance, including being a lead author for the IOC (International Olympic Committee) consensus meeting in nutrition. Trent has attended over ten World or Olympic championships as a nutrition and physiology expert as part of the Canadian integrated support team.

TRAINING —— PLANS AND —— PACE TABLES

"Our goals can only be reached
through a vehicle of a plan, in which
we must fervently believe, and which
we must vigorously act. There is no
other route to success."

— Pablo Picasso

CHAPTER 17

SMT 20-WEEK TRAINING

Note: Just 3 reps of lunges on each side this week for all LMLS warm-ups.

M LMLS, 45 minutes easy with 5 x 20 second strides (60-90 seconds easy recovery), SAM Easy.

T LMLS, 10-minute warm-up, 30 minutes of 3 minutes on, 2 minutes steady fartlek, 10-minute cool-down, SAM Hard.

W LMLS, 50 minutes easy, SAM Easy.

Th LMLS, 45 minutes easy cross training, SAM Easy.

F LMLS, 40 minutes easy with 5 x 20 second strides (60-90 seconds easy recovery), SAM Easy.

S LMLS, 10 miles easy, then immediately into SAM Hard.

Su Brisk walk of 45-60 minutes, LMLS before and SAM Easy afterward is encouraged.

WEEK 1

Note: Just 4 reps of lunges on each side this week for all LMLS warm-ups.

M LMLS, 45 minutes easy with 5 x 20 second strides (60-90 seconds easy recovery), SAM Easy.

T LMLS, 10-minute warm-up, 30-minute progression run: 10 minutes steady, 10 minutes faster, 5 minutes faster, 5 minutes fastest but controlled,10-minute cool-down, SAM Hard.

W LMLS, 55 minutes easy, SAM Easy.

Th LMLS, 45-50 minutes easy cross training, SAM Easy.

F LMLS, 40 minutes easy with 5 x 20 second strides (60-90 seconds easy recovery), SAM Easy.

S LMLS, 11 miles easy, then immediately into SAM Hard.

Su Brisk walk of 45 to 60 minutes, LMLS before and SAM Easy afterward is encouraged.

WEEK 2

WEEK 3

Note: 5 reps of lunges on each side this week for all LMLS warm-ups. This is the full LM warm-up.

M   LMLS, 50 minutes easy with 5 x 20 second strides (60-90 seconds easy recovery), SAM Easy.

T   LMLS, 10-minute warm-up, 4 x 8 minutes at a challenging pace with 3-minute steady recoveries, 10-minute cool-down, SAM Hard.

W   LMLS, 60 minutes easy, SAM Easy.

Th   LMLS, 45-50 minutes easy cross training, SAM Easy.

F   LMLS, 45 minutes easy with 5 x 20 second strides (60-90 seconds easy recovery), SAM Easy.

S   LMLS, 12 miles easy, then immediately into SAM Hard.

Su   Brisk walk of 50 to 65 minutes, LMLS before and SAM Easy afterward is encouraged.

WEEK 4

M   LMLS, 50 minutes easy with 5 x 20 second strides (60-90 seconds easy recovery), SAM Easy.

T   LMLS, 10-minute warm-up, 20 minutes of 3 minutes on, 2 minutes steady, right into 20 minutes of 4 minutes on, 1-minute steady, 10-minute cool-down, SAM Hard.

W   LMLS, 60-65 minutes easy, SAM Easy.

Th   LMLS, 45 minutes easy cross training, SAM Easy. Note: Must make sure the cross training is easy today.

F   Pre-race, LMLS, 10-15 minutes easy, 4-5 x 20 second strides (60-90 seconds easy recovery) 5-minute cool-down.

S   Pre-race, LMLS, 10-15 minutes easy, 4-5 x 20 second strides, finishing the strides roughly a minute or two before the gun goes off. Execute a great 5k Race! 10-minute cool-down down jog, then SAM Easy after the race.

Su   Brisk walk of 35 to 60 minutes, LMLS before and SAM Easy afterward is encouraged.

WEEK 5

M Day off - no running or cross training. If you must do something you can do the mobility work from SAM and you can do rope stretching.

T LMLS, 60 minutes easy cross training, SAM Easy.

W LMLS, 45 minutes easy, SAM Easy.

Th LMLS, 45-55 minutes easy cross training, SAM Easy.

F LMLS, 45 minutes easy with 5 x 20 second strides (60-90 seconds easy recovery), SAM Easy.

S LMLS, 13 miles easy, then immediately into SAM Hard.

Su Brisk walk of 60 to 75 minutes, LMLS before and SAM Easy afterward is encouraged.

WEEK 6

Note: Strides are now 25 seconds per stride.

M LMLS, 50 minutes easy with 5 x 25 second strides (60-90 seconds easy recovery), SAM Easy.

T Pre-race warm-up, Yasso 800s - 8 x 800m with 400m jog, 10-minute cool-down jog, then SAM Hard.

W LMLS, 60-minute easy run, SAM Easy.

Th LMLS, 45-60 minutes easy cross training, SAM Easy.

F LMLS, 45-50 minutes easy with 5 x 25 second strides (60-90 seconds easy recovery), SAM Easy.

S LMLS, 14 miles easy, then immediately into SAM Hard.

Su Brisk walk of 60 to 80 minutes, LMLS before and SAM Easy afterward is encouraged.

WEEK 7

M	LMLS, 55 minutes easy with 5 x 25 second strides (60-90 seconds easy recovery), SAM Easy.
T	LMLS, 10-minute warm-up, 45 minutes of 4 minutes on, 1 minute steady fartlek, 10-minute cool-down, SAM Hard.
W	LMLS, 60-70 minutes easy running, SAM Easy.
Th	LMLS, 45-60 minutes easy cross training, SAM Easy.
F	LMLS, 55 minutes easy with 5 x 25 second strides (60-90 seconds easy recovery), SAM Easy.
S	LMLS, 14 miles easy and if you feel good, at the 11-mile mark you can speed up a bit in the last 3 miles, then immediately into SAM Hard.
Su	Brisk walk of 60 to 85 minutes, LMLS before and SAM Easy afterward is encouraged.

WEEK 8

M	LMLS, 55 minutes easy with 5 x 25 second strides (60-90 seconds easy recovery), SAM Easy.
T	LMLS, 10-minute warm-up, 50 minute progression run: 20 minutes steady, 15 minutes faster, 10 minutes faster, 5 minutes fastest but controlled, 10-minute cool-down, SAM Hard.
W	LMLS, 60-75 minutes easy, SAM Easy.
Th	LMLS, 45-60 minutes easy cross training, SAM Easy.
F	LMLS, 55 minutes easy with 5 x 25 second strides (60-90 seconds easy recovery), SAM Easy.
S	LMLS, 16 miles easy, then immediately into SAM Hard.
Su	Brisk walk of 60-90 minutes, LMLS before and SAM Easy afterward is encouraged.

WEEK 9

Note: Strides are now 30 seconds per stride.

M   LMLS, 55 minutes easy with 5 x 30 second strides (60-90 seconds easy recovery), SAM Easy.

T   LMLS, 10-minute warm-up, 4 x 8 minutes at a challenging pace with 3-minute steady recoveries, 10-minute cool-down, SAM Hard.

W   LMLS, 60-80 minutes easy, SAM Easy.

Th   LMLS, 45-60 minutes easy cross training, SAM Easy.

F   LMLS, 55 minutes easy with 5 x 30 second strides (60-90 seconds easy recovery), SAM Easy.

S   LMLS, 16 miles easy and if you feel good, at the 13-mile mark you can speed up a bit in the last 3 miles, then immediately into SAM Hard.

Su   Brisk walk of 60-85 minutes, LMLS before and SAM Easy afterward is encouraged.

WEEK 10

M   LMLS, 55 minutes easy with 5 x 30 second strides (60-90 seconds easy recovery), SAM Easy.

T   Pre-race warm-up, Yasso 800s - 9 x 800m with 400m jog, 10-minute cool-down jog, then SAM Hard.

W   LMLS, 60-70 minutes easy, SAM Easy.

Th   LMLS, 45-60 minutes easy cross training, SAM Easy.

F   LMLS, 55 minutes easy with 5 x 30 second strides (60-90 seconds easy recovery), SAM Easy.

S   LMLS, 18 miles easy then immediately into SAM Hard after the run.

Su   Brisk walk of 60-85 minutes, LMLS before and SAM Easy afterward is encouraged.

WEEK 11

M	LMLS, 55 minutes easy with 5 x 30 second strides (60-90 seconds easy recovery), SAM Easy.
T	LMLS, 10-minute warm-up, 50 minute progression run: 20 minutes steady, 15 minutes faster, 10 minutes faster, 5 minutes fastest but controlled, 10-minute cool-down, SAM Hard.
W	LMLS, 60-85 minutes easy, SAM Easy.
Th	LMLS, 45-60 minutes easy cross training, SAM Easy.
F	LMLS, 55 minutes easy with 5 x 30 second strides (60-90 seconds easy recovery), SAM Easy.
S	LMLS, 18 miles easy and if you feel good, at the 15-mile mark you can speed up a bit in the last 3 miles, then immediately into SAM Hard.
Su	Brisk walk of 60-90 minutes, LMLS before and SAM Easy afterward is encouraged.

WEEK 12

M	LMLS, 55 minutes easy with 5 x 30 second strides (60-90 seconds easy recovery), SAM Easy.
T	LMLS, 10-minute warm-up, 5 x 8 minutes at a challenging pace with 2-minute slow recoveries, 10-minute cool-down, SAM Hard.
W	LMLS, 60-90 minutes easy, SAM Easy.
Th	LMLS, 45-60 minutes easy cross training, SAM Easy.
F	LMLS, 50 minutes easy with 5 x 30 second strides (60-90 seconds easy recovery), SAM Easy.
S	LMLS, 20 miles easy then immediately into SAM Hard after the run.
Su	Brisk walk of 60-90 minutes, LMLS before and SAM Easy afterward is encouraged.

WEEK 13

M   LMLS, 55 minutes easy with 5 x 30 second strides (60-90 seconds easy recovery), SAM Easy.

T   LMLS, 10-minute warm-up, 60 minute progression run: 30 minutes steady, 15 minutes faster, 10 minutes faster, 5 minutes fastest but controlled, 10-minute cool-down, SAM Hard.

W   LMLS, 60-90 minutes easy, SAM Easy.

Th LMLS, 45-60 minutes of easy cross training, SAM Easy.

F   LMLS, 55 minutes easy with 5 x 30 second strides (60-90 seconds easy recovery), SAM Easy.

S   LMLS, 18 miles easy and if you feel good, at the 14-mile mark you can speed up a bit in the last 4 miles, then immediately into SAM Hard.

Su Brisk walk of 60-90 minutes, LMLS before and SAM Easy afterward is encouraged.

WEEK 14

M   LMLS, 55 minutes easy with 5 x 30 second strides (60-90 seconds easy recovery), SAM Easy.

T   Pre-race warm-up, Yasso 800s - 10 x 800m with 400m jog, 10 minute cool-down jog, then SAM Hard.

W   LMLS, 60 minutes easy, SAM Easy.

Th LMLS, 45-60 minutes easy cross training, SAM Easy.

F   LMLS, 50 minutes easy with 5 x 30 second strides (60-90 seconds easy recovery), SAM Easy.

S   LMLS, 20 miles easy and if you feel good, at the 17-mile mark you can speed up a bit in the last 3 miles, then immediately into SAM Hard.

Su Brisk walk of 60-90 minutes, LMLS before and SAM Easy afterward is encouraged.

M	LMLS, 55 minutes easy with 5 x 30 second strides (60-90 seconds easy recovery), SAM Easy.
T	LMLS, 2 miles warm-up, 4 miles at MP, 1 mile at HMP, 3 miles at MP, 1 mile cool-down, SAM Hard.
W	LMLS, 60-90 minutes easy, SAM Easy.
Th	LMLS, 45-60 minutes easy cross training, SAM Easy.
F	LMLS, 50 minutes easy with 5 x 30 second strides (60-90 seconds easy recovery), SAM Easy.
S	LMLS, 18 miles easy, and if you feel good, run 6 miles at MP from mile 11 to mile 17, finishing with 1 mile easy, then immediately into SAM Hard.
Su	Brisk walk of 60-90 minutes, LMLS before and SAM Easy afterward is encouraged.

M	LMLS, 50 minutes easy with 5 x 30 second strides (60-90 seconds easy recovery), SAM Easy.
T	LMLS, 10-minute warm-up, 40 minutes at MP then 5 minutes "fun-fast," finishing with 15 minutes at MP, 10-minute cool-down, then SAM Hard.
W	LMLS, 60 minutes easy, SAM Easy.
Th	LMLS, 35-50 minutes easy cross training, SAM Easy.
F	LMLS, 40 minutes easy with 5 x 30 second strides (60-90 seconds easy recovery), SAM Easy.
S	LMLS, 22 miles easy, the longest run of the training cycle, making sure to run the first 10 miles conservatively, then SAM Easy (not SAM Hard).
Su	Brisk walk of 60-90 minutes, LMLS before and SAM Easy afterward is encouraged. Also, 20-30 minutes of easy walking in the evening is encouraged.

WEEK 17

M   Complete day off from running and cross training.

T   LMLS, 45 minutes easy with 5 x 30 second strides (60-90 seconds easy recovery), SAM Easy.

W   LMLS, 60-70 minutes easy, SAM Easy.

Th   LMLS, 45-60 minutes easy cross training, SAM Easy.

F   LMLS, 50 minutes easy with 5 x 30 second strides (60-90 seconds easy recovery), SAM Easy.

S   LMLS, 16 mile long run: 7 miles easy, 8 miles at MP, 1 mile cool-down, then immediately into SAM Hard.

Su   Brisk walk of 60-90 minutes, LMLS before and SAM Easy afterward is encouraged.

WEEK 18

M   LMLS, 55 minutes with 5 x 30 second strides (60-90 seconds easy recovery), SAM Easy.

T   LMLS, 2 miles warm-up, 4 miles at MP, 1 mile at HMP, 3 miles at MP, 1 mile cool-down, SAM Hard.

W   LMLS, 60-70 minutes easy, SAM Easy.

Th   LMLS, 45-60 minutes easy cross training, SAM Easy.

F   LMLS, 45-50 minutes easy with 5 x 30 second strides (60-90 seconds easy recovery), SAM Easy.

S   LMLS, 14 mile long run: 6 miles easy, 7 miles at MP, 1 mile cool-down, SAM Hard immediately after the run.

Su   Brisk walk of 60 minutes, LMLS before and SAM Easy afterward is encouraged.

WEEK 19

Note: SAM Easy for men on Saturday; SAM Hard for women on Saturday.

M LMLS, 50 minutes easy with 5 x 30 second strides (60-90 seconds easy recovery), SAM Easy.

T LMLS, 2 miles warm-up, 3 miles at MP, 0.5 miles "fun-fast," 3 miles at MP, 1 mile cool-down SAM Hard.

W LMLS, 60 minutes easy, SAM Easy.

Th LMLS, 45 minutes easy cross training, SAM Easy.

F LMLS, 45 minutes easy with 5 x 30 second strides (60-90 seconds easy recovery), SAM Easy.

S LMLS, 12 mile long run: 5 miles easy, 6 miles at MP, 1 mile cool-down, SAM immediately after the run (SAM Easy for men, SAM Hard for women).

Su Brisk walk of 45 minutes, LMLS before and SAM Easy afterward is encouraged.

WEEK 20

M LMLS, 40 minutes easy with 5 x 30 second strides (60-90 seconds easy recovery), SAM Easy.

T LMLS, 1 mile warm-up, 2 miles at MP, 1 mile at HMP, 3 miles at MP, 1 mile cool-down, SAM Easy.

W LMLS, 35-40 minutes easy with 5 x 30 second strides (60-90 seconds easy recovery), SAM Easy.

Th Complete day off from running and cross training.

F LMLS, 30-35 minutes easy, SAM Easy.

S Pre-race, 10-15 minute easy running, then 5 x 30 second strides (60-90 seconds easy recovery), then 5-minute cool-down, LS and hip mobility from Phase 1 SAM Easy.

Su Race! Execute a smart race plan and you'll be happy with the result. Remember, be conservative in the opening miles of the race.

YASSO 800M WORKOUT/
MARATHON PACE
TABLES

Yasso Avg 800m split	Projected Marathon	Marathon Pace
2:30	2:35	5:54
2:31	2:36	5:56
2:32	2:37	5:59
2:33	2:38	6:01
2:34	2:39	6:03
2:35	2:40	6:06
2:36	2:41	6:08
2:37	2:42	6:10
2:38	2:43	6:13
2:39	2:44	6:15
2:40	2:45	6:17
2:41	2:46	6:19
2:42	2:47	6:22
2:43	2:48	6:24
2:44	2:49	6:26
2:45	2:50	6:29
2:46	2:51	6:31
2:47	2:52	6:33
2:48	2:53	6:35
2:49	2:54	6:38
2:50	2:55	6:40

Yasso Avg 800m split	Projected Marathon	Marathon Pace
2:51	2:56	6:42
2:52	2:57	6:45
2:53	2:58	6:47
2:54	2:59	6:49
2:55	3:00	6:51
2:56	3:01	6:54
2:57	3:02	6:56
2:58	3:03	6:58
2:59	3:04	7:01
3:00	3:05	7:03
3:01	3:06	7:05
3:02	3:07	7:07
3:03	3:08	7:10
3:04	3:09	7:12
3:05	3:10	7:14
3:06	3:11	7:17
3:07	3:12	7:19
3:08	3:13	7:21
3:09	3:14	7:23
3:10	3:15	7:26

Yasso Avg 800m split	Projected Marathon	Marathon Pace
3:11	3:16	7:28
3:12	3:17	7:30
3:13	3:18	7:33
3:14	3:19	7:35
3:15	3:20	7:37
3:16	3:21	7:39
3:17	3:22	7:42
3:18	3:23	7:44
3:19	3:24	7:46
3:20	3:25	7:49
3:21	3:26	7:51
3:22	3:27	7:53
3:23	3:28	7:55
3:24	3:29	7:58
3:25	3:30	8:00
3:26	3:31	8:02
3:27	3:32	8:05
3:28	3:33	8:07
3:29	3:34	8:09
3:30	3:35	8:12
3:31	3:36	8:14
3:32	3:37	8:16
3:33	3:38	8:18
3:34	3:39	8:21
3:35	3:40	8:23

Yasso Avg 800m split	Projected Marathon	Marathon Pace
3:36	3:41	8:25
3:37	3:42	8:28
3:38	3:43	8:30
3:39	3:44	8:32
3:40	3:45	8:34
3:41	3:46	8:37
3:42	3:47	8:39
3:43	3:48	8:41
3:44	3:49	8:44
3:45	3:50	8:46
3:46	3:51	8:48
3:47	3:52	8:50
3:48	3:53	8:53
3:49	3:54	8:55
3:50	3:55	8:57
3:51	3:56	9:00
3:52	3:57	9:02
3:53	3:58	9:04
3:54	3:59	9:06
3:55	4:00	9:09
3:56	4:01	9:11
3:57	4:02	9:13
3:58	4:03	9:16
3:59	4:04	9:18
4:00	4:05	9:20

Yasso Avg 800m split	Projected Marathon	Marathon Pace	Yasso Avg 800m split	Projected Marathon	Marathon Pace
4:01	4:06	9:22	4:26	4:31	10:20
4:02	4:07	9:25	4:27	4:32	10:22
4:03	4:08	9:27	4:28	4:33	10:24
4:04	4:09	9:29	4:29	4:34	10:27
4:05	4:10	9:32	4:30	4:35	10:29
4:06	4:11	9:34	4:31	4:36	10:31
4:07	4:12	9:36	4:32	4:37	10:33
4:08	4:13	9:38	4:33	4:38	10:36
4:09	4:14	9:41	4:34	4:39	10:38
4:10	4:15	9:43	4:35	4:40	10:40
4:11	4:16	9:45	4:36	4:41	10:43
4:12	4:17	9:48	4:37	4:42	10:45
4:13	4:18	9:50	4:38	4:43	10:47
4:14	4:19	9:52	4:39	4:44	10:49
4:15	4:20	9:54	4:40	4:45	10:52
4:16	4:21	9:57	4:41	4:46	10:54
4:17	4:22	9:59	4:42	4:47	10:56
4:18	4:23	10:01	4:43	4:48	10:59
4:19	4:24	10:04	4:44	4:49	11:01
4:20	4:25	10:06	4:45	4:50	11:03
4:21	4:26	10:08	4:46	4:51	11:05
4:22	4:27	10:11	4:47	4:52	11:08
4:23	4:28	10:13	4:48	4:53	11:10
4:24	4:29	10:15	4:49	4:54	11:12
4:25	4:30	10:17	4:50	4:55	11:15

Yasso Avg 800m split	Projected Marathon	Marathon Pace
4:51	4:56	11:17
4:52	4:57	11:19
4:53	4:58	11:21
4:54	4:59	11:24
4:55	5:00	11:26
4:56	5:01	11:28
4:57	5:02	11:31
4:58	5:03	11:33
4:59	5:04	11:35
5:00	5:05	11:37

WEDNESDAY/SUNDAY TRAINING

Note: Just 3 reps of lunges on each side this week for all LMLS warm-ups.

M   Start the SMT System on Tuesday.

T   LMLS, 45 minutes easy with 5 x 20 second strides (60-90 seconds easy recovery), SAM Easy.

W   LMLS, 10-minute warm-up, 30 minutes of 3 minutes on, 2 minutes steady fartlek, 10-minute cool-down, SAM Hard.

Th   LMLS, 50 minutes easy, SAM Easy.

F   LMLS, 45 minutes easy cross training, SAM Easy.

S   LMLS, 40 minutes easy with 5 x 20 second strides (60-90 seconds easy recovery), SAM Easy.

Su   LMLS, 10 miles easy, then immediately into SAM Hard.

Note: Just 4 reps of lunges on each side this week for all LMLS warm-ups.

M   Brisk walk of 45-60 minutes, LMLS before and SAM Easy afterward is encouraged.

T   LMLS, 45 minutes easy with 5 x 20 second strides (60-90 seconds easy recovery), SAM Easy.

W   LMLS, 10-minute warm-up, 30-minute progression run: 10 minutes steady, 10 minutes faster, 5 minutes faster, 5 minutes fastest but controlled,10-minute cool-down, SAM Hard.

Th   LMLS, 55 minutes easy, SAM Easy.

F   LMLS, 45-50 minutes easy cross training, SAM Easy.

S   LMLS, 40 minutes easy with 5 x 20 second strides (60-90 seconds easy recovery), SAM Easy.

Su   LMLS, 11 miles easy, then immediately into SAM Hard.

WEEK 3

Note: 5 reps of lunges on each side this week for all LMLS warm-ups. This is the full LM warm-up.

M   Brisk walk of 45 to 60 minutes, LMLS before and SAM Easy afterward is encouraged.

T   LMLS, 50 minutes easy with 5 x 20 second strides (60-90 seconds easy recovery), SAM Easy.

W   LMLS, 10-minute warm-up, 4 x 8 minutes at a challenging pace with 3-minute steady recoveries, 10-minute cool-down, SAM Hard.

Th   LMLS, 60 minutes easy, SAM Easy.

F   LMLS, 45-50 minutes easy cross training, SAM Easy.

S   LMLS, 45 minutes easy with 5 x 20 second strides (60-90 seconds easy recovery), SAM Easy.

Su   LMLS, 12 miles easy, then immediately into SAM Hard.

WEEK 4

M   Brisk walk of 50 to 65 minutes, LMLS before and SAM Easy afterward is encouraged.

T   LMLS, 50 minutes easy with 5 x 20 second strides (60-90 seconds easy recovery), SAM Easy.

W   LMLS, 10-minute warm-up, 20 minutes of 3 minutes on, 2 minutes steady, right into 20 minutes of 4 minutes on, 1-minute steady, 10-minute cool-down, SAM Hard.

Th   LMLS, 60-65 minutes easy, SAM Easy.

F   LMLS, 45 minutes easy cross training, SAM Easy. Note: Must make sure the cross training is easy today.

S   Pre-race, LMLS, 10-15 minutes easy, 4-5 x 20 second strides (60-90 seconds easy recovery) 5-minute cool-down.

Su   Pre-race, LMLS, 10-15 minutes easy, 4-5 x 20 second strides, finishing the strides roughly a minute or two before the gun goes off. Execute a great 5k Race! 10-minute cool-down down jog, then SAM Easy after the race.

WEEK 5

M   Brisk walk of 35 to 60 minutes, LMLS before and SAM Easy afterward is encouraged.

T   Day off - no running or cross training. If you must do something you can do the mobility work from SAM and you can do rope stretching.

W   LMLS, 60 minutes easy cross training, SAM Easy.

Th LMLS, 45 minutes easy, SAM Easy.

F   LMLS, 45-55 minutes easy cross training, SAM Easy.

S   LMLS, 45 minutes easy with 5 x 20 second strides (60-90 seconds easy recovery), SAM Easy.

Su LMLS, 13 miles easy, then immediately into SAM Hard.

WEEK 6

Note: Strides are now 25 seconds per stride.

M   Brisk walk of 60 to 75 minutes, LMLS before and SAM Easy afterward is encouraged.

T   LMLS, 50 minutes easy with 5 x 25 second strides (60-90 seconds easy recovery), SAM Easy.

W   Pre-race warm-up, Yasso 800s - 8 x 800m with 400m jog, 10 minute cool-down jog, then SAM Hard.

Th LMLS, 60-minute easy run, SAM Easy.

F   LMLS, 45-60 minutes easy cross training, SAM Easy.

S   LMLS, 45-50 minutes easy with 5 x 25 second strides (60-90 seconds easy recovery), SAM Easy.

Su LMLS, 14 miles easy, then immediately into SAM Hard.

WEEK 7

M	Brisk walk of 60 to 80 minutes, LMLS before and SAM Easy afterward is encouraged.
T	LMLS, 55 minutes easy with 5 x 25 second strides (60-90 seconds easy recovery), SAM Easy.
W	LMLS, 10-minute warm-up, 45 minutes of 4 minutes on, 1 minute steady fartlek, 10-minute cool-down, SAM Hard.
Th	LMLS, 60-70 minutes easy running, SAM Easy.
F	LMLS, 45-60 minutes easy cross training, SAM Easy.
S	LMLS, 55 minutes easy with 5 x 25 second strides (60-90 seconds easy recovery), SAM Easy.
Su	LMLS, 14 miles easy and if you feel good, at the 11-mile mark you can speed up a bit in the last 3 miles, then immediately into SAM Hard.

WEEK 8

M	Brisk walk of 60 to 85 minutes, LMLS before and SAM Easy afterward is encouraged.
T	LMLS, 55 minutes easy with 5 x 25 second strides (60-90 seconds easy recovery), SAM Easy.
W	LMLS, 10-minute warm-up, 50 minute progression run: 20 minutes steady, 15 minutes faster, 10 minutes faster, 5 minutes fastest but controlled, 10-minute cool-down, SAM Hard.
Th	LMLS, 60-75 minutes easy, SAM Easy.
F	LMLS, 45-60 minutes easy cross training, SAM Easy.
S	LMLS, 55 minutes easy with 5 x 25 second strides (60-90 seconds easy recovery), SAM Easy.
Su	LMLS, 16 miles easy, then immediately into SAM Hard.

WEEK 9

Note: Strides are now 30 seconds per stride.

M   Brisk walk of 60-90 minutes, LMLS before and SAM Easy afterward is encouraged.

T   LMLS, 55 minutes easy with 5 x 30 second strides (60-90 seconds easy recovery), SAM Easy.

W   LMLS, 10-minute warm-up, 4 x 8 minutes at a challenging pace with 3-minute steady recoveries, 10-minute cool-down, SAM Hard.

Th   LMLS, 60-80 minutes easy, SAM Easy.

F   LMLS, 45-60 minutes easy cross training, SAM Easy.

S   LMLS, 55 minutes easy with 5 x 30 second strides (60-90 seconds easy recovery), SAM Easy.

Su   LMLS, 16 miles easy and if you feel good, at the 13-mile mark you can speed up a bit in the last 3 miles, then immediately into SAM Hard.

WEEK 10

M   Brisk walk of 60-85 minutes, LMLS before and SAM Easy afterward is encouraged.

T   LMLS, 55 minutes easy with 5 x 30 second strides (60-90 seconds easy recovery), SAM Easy.

W   Pre-race warm-up, Yasso 800s - 9 x 800m with 400m jog, 10-minute cool-down jog, then SAM Hard.

Th   LMLS, 60-70 minutes easy, SAM Easy.

F   LMLS, 45-60 minutes easy cross training, SAM Easy.

S   LMLS, 55 minutes easy with 5 x 30 second strides (60-90 seconds easy recovery), SAM Easy.

Su   LMLS, 18 miles easy then immediately into SAM Hard after the run.

WEEK 11

M	Brisk walk of 60-85 minutes, LMLS before and SAM Easy afterward is encouraged.
T	LMLS, 55 minutes easy with 5 x 30 second strides (60-90 seconds easy recovery), SAM Easy.
W	LMLS, 10-minute warm-up, 50 minute progression run: 20 minutes steady, 15 minutes faster, 10 minutes faster, 5 minutes fastest but controlled, 10-minute cool-down, SAM Hard.
Th	LMLS, 60-85 minutes easy, SAM Easy.
F	LMLS, 45-60 minutes easy cross training, SAM Easy.
S	LMLS, 55 minutes easy with 5 x 30 second strides (60-90 seconds easy recovery), SAM Easy.
Su	LMLS, 18 miles easy and if you feel good, at the 15-mile mark you can speed up a bit in the last 3 miles, then immediately into SAM Hard.

WEEK 12

M	Brisk walk of 60-90 minutes, LMLS before and SAM Easy afterward is encouraged.
T	LMLS, 55 minutes easy with 5 x 30 second strides (60-90 seconds easy recovery), SAM Easy.
W	LMLS, 10-minute warm-up, 5 x 8 minutes at a challenging pace with 2-minute slow recoveries, 10-minute cool-down, SAM Hard.
Th	LMLS, 60-90 minutes easy, SAM Easy.
F	LMLS, 45-60 minutes easy cross training, SAM Easy.
S	LMLS, 50 minutes easy with 5 x 30 second strides (60-90 seconds easy recovery), SAM Easy.
Su	LMLS, 20 miles easy then immediately into SAM Hard after the run.

WEEK 13

M   Brisk walk of 60-90 minutes, LMLS before and SAM Easy afterward is encouraged.

T   LMLS, 55 minutes easy with 5 x 30 second strides (60-90 seconds easy recovery), SAM Easy.

W   LMLS, 10-minute warm-up, 60 minute progression run: 30 minutes steady, 15 minutes faster, 10 minutes faster, 5 minutes fastest but controlled, 10-minute cool-down, SAM Hard.

Th LMLS, 60-90 minutes easy, SAM Easy.

F   LMLS, 45-60 minutes of easy cross training, SAM Easy.

S   LMLS, 55 minutes easy with 5 x 30 second strides (60-90 seconds easy recovery), SAM Easy.

Su LMLS, 18 miles easy and if you feel good, at the 14-mile mark you can speed up a bit in the last 4 miles, then immediately into SAM Hard.

WEEK 14

M   Brisk walk of 60-90 minutes, LMLS before and SAM Easy afterward is encouraged.

T   LMLS, 55 minutes easy with 5 x 30 second strides (60-90 seconds easy recovery), SAM Easy.

W   Pre-race warm-up, Yasso 800s - 10 x 800m with 400m jog, 10 minute cool-down jog, then SAM Hard.

Th LMLS, 60 minutes easy, SAM Easy.

F   LMLS, 45-60 minutes easy cross training, SAM Easy.

S   LMLS, 50 minutes easy with 5 x 30 second strides (60-90 seconds easy recovery), SAM Easy.

Su LMLS, 20 miles easy and if you feel good, at the 17-mile mark you can speed up a bit in the last 3 miles, then immediately into SAM Hard.

WEEK 15

M	Brisk walk of 60-90 minutes, LMLS before and SAM Easy afterward is encouraged.
T	LMLS, 55 minutes easy with 5 x 30 second strides (60-90 seconds easy recovery), SAM Easy.
W	LMLS, 2 miles warm-up, 4 miles at MP, 1 mile at HMP, 3 miles at MP, 1 mile cool-down, SAM Hard.
Th	LMLS, 60-90 minutes easy, SAM Easy.
F	LMLS, 45-60 minutes easy cross training, SAM Easy.
S	LMLS, 50 minutes easy with 5 x 30 second strides (60-90 seconds easy recovery), SAM Easy.
Su	LMLS, 18 miles easy, and if you feel good, run 6 miles at MP from mile 11 to mile 17, finishing with 1 mile easy, then immediately into SAM Hard.

WEEK 16

M	Brisk walk of 60-90 minutes, LMLS before and SAM Easy afterward is encouraged.
T	LMLS, 50 minutes easy with 5 x 30 second strides (60-90 seconds easy recovery), SAM Easy.
W	LMLS, 10-minute warm-up, 40 minutes at MP then 5 minutes "fun-fast," finishing with 15 minutes at MP, 10-minute cool-down, then SAM Hard.
Th	LMLS, 60 minutes easy, SAM Easy.
F	LMLS, 35-50 minutes easy cross training, SAM Easy.
S	LMLS, 40 minutes easy with 5 x 30 second strides (60-90 seconds easy recovery), SAM Easy.
Su	LMLS, 22 miles easy, the longest run of the training cycle, making sure to run the first 10 miles conservatively, then SAM Easy (not SAM Hard).

M   Brisk walk of 60-90 minutes, LMLS before and SAM Easy afterward is encouraged. Also, 20-30 minutes of easy walking in the evening is encouraged.

T   Complete day off from running and cross training.

W   LMLS, 45 minutes easy with 5 x 30 second strides (60-90 seconds easy recovery), SAM Easy.

Th LMLS, 60-70 minutes easy, SAM Easy.

F   LMLS, 45-60 minutes easy cross training, SAM Easy.

S   LMLS, 50 minutes easy with 5 x 30 second strides (60-90 seconds easy recovery), SAM Easy.

Su LMLS, 16 mile long run: 7 miles easy, 8 miles at MP, 1 mile cool-down, then immediately into SAM Hard.

M   Brisk walk of 60-90 minutes, LMLS before and SAM Easy afterward is encouraged.

T   LMLS, 55 minutes with 5 x 30 second strides (60-90 seconds easy recovery), SAM Easy.

W   LMLS, 2 miles warm-up, 4 miles at MP, 1 mile at HMP, 3 miles at MP, 1 mile cool-down, SAM Hard.

Th LMLS, 60-70 minutes easy, SAM Easy.

F   LMLS, 45-60 minutes easy cross training, SAM Easy.

S   LMLS, 45-50 minutes easy with 5 x 30 second strides (60-90 seconds easy recovery), SAM Easy.

Su LMLS, 14 mile long run: 6 miles easy, 7 miles at MP, 1 mile cool-down, SAM Hard immediately after the run.

WEEK 19

Note: SAM Easy for men on Saturday; SAM Hard for women on Saturday.

M   Brisk walk of 60 minutes, LMLS before and SAM Easy afterward is encouraged.

T   LMLS, 50 minutes easy with 5 x 30 second strides (60-90 seconds easy recovery), SAM Easy.

W   LMLS, 2 miles warm-up, 3 miles at MP, 0.5 miles "fun-fast," 3 miles at MP, 1 mile cool-down SAM Hard.

Th LMLS, 60 minutes easy, SAM Easy.

F   LMLS, 45 minutes easy cross training, SAM Easy.

S   LMLS, 45 minutes easy with 5 x 30 second strides (60-90 seconds easy recovery), SAM Easy.

Su LMLS, 12 mile long run: 5 miles easy, 6 miles at MP, 1 mile cool-down, SAM immediately after the run (SAM Easy for men, SAM Hard for women).

WEEK 20

M   Brisk walk of 45 minutes, LMLS before and SAM Easy afterward is encouraged.

T   LMLS, 1 mile warm-up, 2 miles at MP, 1 mile at HMP, 3 miles at MP, 1 mile cool-down, SAM Easy.

W   LMLS, 35-40 minutes easy with 5 x 30 second strides (60-90 seconds easy recovery), SAM Easy.

Th Complete day off from running and cross training.

F   LMLS, 30-35 minutes easy, SAM Easy.

S   Pre-race, 10-15 minute easy running, then 5 x 30 second strides (60-90 seconds easy recovery), then 5-minute cool-down, LS and hip mobility from Phase 1 SAM Easy.

Su Race! Execute a smart race plan and you'll be happy with the result. Remember, be conservative in the opening miles of the race.

MONDAY/FRIDAY TRAINING

Note: Just 3 reps of lunges on each side this week for all LMLS warm-ups.

WEEK 1

M LMLS, 10-minute warm-up, 30 minutes of 3 minutes on, 2 minutes steady fartlek, 10-minute cool-down, SAM Hard.

T LMLS, 50 minutes easy, SAM Easy.

W LMLS, 45 minutes easy cross training, SAM Easy.

Th LMLS, 40 minutes easy with 5 x 20 second strides (60-90 seconds easy recovery), SAM Easy.

F LMLS, 10 miles easy, then immediately into SAM Hard.

S Brisk walk of 45-60 minutes, LMLS before and SAM Easy afterward is encouraged.

Su LMLS, 45 minutes easy with 5 x 20 second strides (60-90 seconds easy recovery), SAM Easy.

Note: Just 4 reps of lunges on each side this week for all LMLS warm-ups.

WEEK 2

M LMLS, 10-minute warm-up, 30-minute progression run: 10 minutes steady, 10 minutes faster, 5 minutes faster, 5 minutes fastest but controlled,10-minute cool-down, SAM Hard.

T LMLS, 55 minutes easy, SAM Easy.

W LMLS, 45-50 minutes easy cross training, SAM Easy.

Th LMLS, 40 minutes easy with 5 x 20 second strides (60-90 seconds easy recovery), SAM Easy.

F LMLS, 11 miles easy, then immediately into SAM Hard.

S Brisk walk of 45 to 60 minutes, LMLS before and SAM Easy afterward is encouraged.

Su LMLS, 50 minutes easy with 5 x 20 second strides (60-90 seconds easy recovery), SAM Easy.

Note: 5 reps of lunges on each side this week for all LMLS warm-ups. This is the full LM warm-up.

WEEK 3

M   LMLS, 10-minute warm-up, 4 x 8 minutes at a challenging pace with 3-minute steady recoveries, 10-minute cool-down, SAM Hard.

T   LMLS, 60 minutes easy, SAM Easy.

W   LMLS, 45-50 minutes easy cross training, SAM Easy.

Th   LMLS, 45 minutes easy with 5 x 20 second strides (60-90 seconds easy recovery), SAM Easy.

F   LMLS, 12 miles easy, then immediately into SAM Hard.

S   Brisk walk of 50 to 65 minutes, LMLS before and SAM Easy afterward is encouraged.

Su   LMLS, 50 minutes easy with 5 x 20 second strides (60-90 seconds easy recovery), SAM Easy.

WEEK 4

M   LMLS, 10-minute warm-up, 20 minutes of 3 minutes on, 2 minutes steady, right into 20 minutes of 4 minutes on, 1-minute steady, 10-minute cool-down, SAM Hard.

T   LMLS, 60-65 minutes easy, SAM Easy.

W   LMLS, 45 minutes easy cross training, SAM Easy. Note: Must make sure the cross training is easy today.

Th   LMLS, 35 minutes with 5 x 20 second strides (60-90 seconds easy recovery), SAM Easy.

F   Pre-race, LMLS, 10-15 minutes easy, 4-5 x 20 second strides (60-90 seconds easy recovery) 5-minute cool-down.

S   Pre-race, LMLS, 10-15 minutes easy, 4-5 x 20 second strides, finishing the strides roughly a minute or two before the gun goes off. Execute a great 5k Race! 10-minute cool-down down jog, then SAM Easy after the race.

Su   Brisk walk of 35 to 60 minutes, LMLS before and SAM Easy afterward is encouraged.

WEEK 5

M   Day off – no running or cross training. If you must do something you can do the mobility work from SAM and you can do rope stretching.

T   LMLS, 60 minutes easy cross training, SAM Easy.

W   LMLS, 45 minutes easy, SAM Easy.

Th   LMLS, 45 minutes easy with 5 x 20 second strides (60-90 seconds easy recovery), SAM Easy.

F   LMLS, 13 miles easy, then immediately into SAM Hard.

S   Brisk walk of 60 to 75 minutes, LMLS before and SAM Easy afterward is encouraged.

Su   LMLS, 50 minutes easy with 5 x 25 second strides (60-90 seconds easy recovery), SAM Easy.

WEEK 6

Note: Strides are now 25 seconds per stride.

M   Pre-race warm-up, Yasso 800s – 8 x 800m with 400m jog, 10 minute cool-down jog, then SAM Hard.

T   LMLS, 60-minute easy run, SAM Easy.

W   LMLS, 45-60 minutes easy cross training, SAM Easy.

Th   LMLS, 45-50 minutes easy with 5 x 25 second strides (60-90 seconds easy recovery), SAM Easy.

F   LMLS, 14 miles easy, then immediately into SAM Hard.

S   Brisk walk of 60 to 80 minutes, LMLS before and SAM Easy afterward is encouraged.

Su   LMLS, 55 minutes easy with 5 x 25 second strides (60-90 seconds easy recovery), SAM Easy.

WEEK 7

M LMLS, 10-minute warm-up, 45 minutes of 4 minutes on, 1 minute steady fartlek, 10-minute cool-down, SAM Hard.

T LMLS, 60-70 minutes easy running, SAM Easy.

W LMLS, 45-60 minutes easy cross training, SAM Easy.

Th LMLS, 55 minutes easy with 5 x 25 second strides (60-90 seconds easy recovery), SAM Easy.

F LMLS, 14 miles easy and if you feel good, at the 11-mile mark you can speed up a bit in the last 3 miles, then immediately into SAM Hard.

S Brisk walk of 60 to 85 minutes, LMLS before and SAM Easy afterward is encouraged.

Su LMLS, 55 minutes easy with 5 x 25 second strides (60-90 seconds easy recovery), SAM Easy.

WEEK 8

M LMLS, 10-minute warm-up, 50 minute progression run: 20 minutes steady, 15 minutes faster, 10 minutes faster, 5 minutes fastest but controlled, 10-minute cool-down, SAM Hard.

T LMLS, 60-75 minutes easy, SAM Easy.

W LMLS, 45-60 minutes easy cross training, SAM Easy.

Th LMLS, 55 minutes easy with 5 x 25 second strides (60-90 seconds easy recovery), SAM Easy.

F LMLS, 16 miles easy, then immediately into SAM Hard.

S Brisk walk of 60-90 minutes, LMLS before and SAM Easy afterward is encouraged.

Su LMLS, 55 minutes easy with 5 x 30 second strides (60-90 seconds easy recovery), SAM Easy.

WEEK 9

Note: Strides are now 30 seconds per stride.

M   LMLS, 10-minute warm-up, 4 x 8 minutes at a challenging pace with 3 minute steady recoveries, 10-minute cool-down, SAM Hard.

T   LMLS, 60-80 minutes easy, SAM Easy.

W   LMLS, 45-60 minutes easy cross training, SAM Easy.

Th   LMLS, 55 minutes easy with 5 x 30 second strides (60-90 seconds easy recovery), SAM Easy.

F   LMLS, 16 miles easy and if you feel good, at the 13-mile mark you can speed up a bit in the last 3 miles, then immediately into SAM Hard.

S   Brisk walk of 60-85 minutes, LMLS before and SAM Easy afterward is encouraged.

Su   LMLS, 55 minutes easy with 5 x 30 second strides (60-90 seconds easy recovery), SAM Easy.

WEEK 10

M   Pre-race warm-up, Yasso 800s - 9 x 800m with 400m jog, 10-minute cool-down jog, then SAM Hard.

T   LMLS, 60-70 minutes easy, SAM Easy.

W   LMLS, 45-60 minutes easy cross training, SAM Easy.

Th   LMLS, 55 minutes easy with 5 x 30 second strides (60-90 seconds easy recovery), SAM Easy.

F   LMLS, 18 miles easy then immediately into SAM Hard after the run.

S   Brisk walk of 60-85 minutes, LMLS before and SAM Easy afterward is encouraged.

Su   LMLS, 55 minutes easy with 5 x 30 second strides (60-90 seconds easy recovery), SAM Easy.

WEEK 11

M	LMLS, 10-minute warm-up, 50 minute progression run: 20 minutes steady, 15 minutes faster, 10 minutes faster, 5 minutes fastest but controlled, 10-minute cool-down, SAM Hard.
T	LMLS, 60-85 minutes easy, SAM Easy.
W	LMLS, 45-60 minutes easy cross training, SAM Easy.
Th	LMLS, 55 minutes easy with 5 x 30 second strides (60-90 seconds easy recovery), SAM Easy.
F	LMLS, 18 miles easy and if you feel good, at the 15-mile mark you can speed up a bit in the last 3 miles, then immediately into SAM Hard.
S	Brisk walk of 60-90 minutes, LMLS before and SAM Easy afterward is encouraged.
Su	LMLS, 55 minutes easy with 5 x 30 second strides (60-90 seconds easy recovery), SAM Easy.

WEEK 12

M	LMLS, 10-minute warm-up, 5 x 8 minutes at a challenging pace with 2 minute slow recoveries, 10-minute cool-down, SAM Hard.
T	LMLS, 60-90 minutes easy, SAM Easy.
W	LMLS, 45-60 minutes easy cross training, SAM Easy.
Th	LMLS, 50 minutes easy with 5 x 30 second strides (60-90 seconds easy recovery), SAM Easy.
F	LMLS, 20 miles easy then immediately into SAM Hard after the run.
S	Brisk walk of 60-90 minutes, LMLS before and SAM Easy afterward is encouraged.
Su	LMLS, 55 minutes easy with 5 x 30 second strides (60-90 seconds easy recovery), SAM Easy.

WEEK 13

M   LMLS, 10-minute warm-up, 60 minute progression run: 30 minutes steady, 15 minutes faster, 10 minutes faster, 5 minutes fastest but controlled, 10-minute cool-down, SAM Hard.

T   LMLS, 60-90 minutes easy, SAM Easy.

W   LMLS, 45-60 minutes of easy cross training, SAM Easy.

Th LMLS, 55 minutes easy with 5 x 30 second strides (60-90 seconds easy recovery), SAM Easy.

F   LMLS, 18 miles easy and if you feel good, at the 14-mile mark you can speed up a bit in the last 4 miles, then immediately into SAM Hard.

S   Brisk walk of 60-90 minutes, LMLS before and SAM Easy afterward is encouraged.

Su LMLS, 55 minutes easy with 5 x 30 second strides (60-90 seconds easy recovery), SAM Easy.

WEEK 14

M   Pre-race warm-up, Yasso 800s - 10 x 800m with 400m jog, 10 minute cool-down jog, then SAM Hard.

T   LMLS, 60 minutes easy, SAM Easy.

W   LMLS, 45-60 minutes easy cross training, SAM Easy.

Th LMLS, 50 minutes easy with 5 x 30 second strides (60-90 seconds easy recovery), SAM Easy.

F   LMLS, 20 miles easy and if you feel good, at the 17-mile mark you can speed up a bit in the last 3 miles, then immediately into SAM Hard.

S   Brisk walk of 60-90 minutes, LMLS before and SAM Easy afterward is encouraged.

Su LMLS, 55 minutes easy with 5 x 30 second strides (60-90 seconds easy recovery), SAM Easy.

WEEK 15

M   LMLS, 2 miles warm-up, 4 miles at MP, 1 mile at HMP, 3 miles at MP, 1 mile cool-down, SAM Hard.

T   LMLS, 60-90 minutes easy, SAM Easy.

W   LMLS, 45-60 minutes easy cross training, SAM Easy.

Th LMLS, 50 minutes easy with 5 x 30 second strides (60-90 seconds easy recovery), SAM Easy.

F   LMLS, 18 miles easy, and if you feel good, run 6 miles at MP from mile 11 to mile 17, finishing with 1 mile easy, then immediately into SAM Hard.

S   Brisk walk of 60-90 minutes, LMLS before and SAM Easy afterward is encouraged.

Su LMLS, 50 minutes easy with 5 x 30 second strides (60-90 seconds easy recovery), SAM Easy.

WEEK 16

M   LMLS, 10-minute warm-up, 40 minutes at MP then 5 minutes "fun-fast," finishing with 15 minutes at MP, 10-minute cool-down, then SAM Hard.

T   LMLS, 60 minutes easy, SAM Easy.

W   LMLS, 35-50 minutes easy cross training, SAM Easy.

Th LMLS, 40 minutes easy with 5 x 30 second strides (60-90 seconds easy recovery), SAM Easy.

F   LMLS, 22 miles easy, the longest run of the training cycle, making sure to run the first 10 miles conservatively, then SAM Easy (not SAM Hard).

S   Brisk walk of 60-90 minutes, LMLS before and SAM Easy afterward is encouraged. Also, 20-30 minutes of easy walking in the evening is encouraged.

Su Complete day off from running and cross training.

WEEK 17

M   LMLS, 45 minutes easy with 5 x 30 second strides (60-90 seconds easy recovery), SAM Easy.

T   LMLS, 60-70 minutes easy, SAM Easy.

W   LMLS, 45-60 minutes easy cross training, SAM Easy.

Th   LMLS, 50 minutes easy with 5 x 30 second strides (60-90 seconds easy recovery), SAM Easy.

F   LMLS, 16 mile long run: 7 miles easy, 8 miles at MP, 1 mile cool-down, then immediately into SAM Hard.

S   Brisk walk of 60-90 minutes, LMLS before and SAM Easy afterward is encouraged.

Su   LMLS, 55 minutes with 5 x 30 second strides (60-90 seconds easy recovery), SAM Easy.

WEEK 18

M   LMLS, 2 miles warm-up, 4 miles at MP, 1 mile at HMP, 3 miles at MP, 1 mile cool-down, SAM Hard.

T   LMLS, 60-70 minutes easy, SAM Easy.

W   LMLS, 45-60 minutes easy cross training, SAM Easy.

Th   LMLS, 45-50 minutes easy with 5 x 30 second strides (60-90 seconds easy recovery), SAM Easy.

F   LMLS, 14 mile long run: 6 miles easy, 7 miles at MP, 1 mile cool-down, SAM Hard immediately after the run.

S   Brisk walk of 60 minutes, LMLS before and SAM Easy afterward is encouraged.

Su   LMLS, 50 minutes easy with 5 x 30 second strides (60-90 seconds easy recovery), SAM Easy.

WEEK 19

Note: SAM Easy for men on Saturday; SAM Hard for women on Saturday.

M   LMLS, 2 miles warm-up, 3 miles at MP, 0.5 miles "fun-fast," 3 miles at MP, 1 mile cool-down SAM Hard.

T   LMLS, 60 minutes easy, SAM Easy.

W   LMLS, 45 minutes easy cross training, SAM Easy.

Th LMLS, 45 minutes easy with 5 x 30 second strides (60-90 seconds easy recovery), SAM Easy.

F   LMLS, 12 mile long run: 5 miles easy, 6 miles at MP, 1 mile cool-down, SAM immediately after the run (SAM Easy for men, SAM Hard for women).

S   Brisk walk of 45 minutes, LMLS before and SAM Easy afterward is encouraged.

Su Complete day off from running and cross training.

WEEK 20

M   LMLS, 35-40 minutes easy with 5 x 30 second strides (60-90 seconds easy recovery), SAM Easy.

T   LMLS, 1 mile warm-up, 2 miles at MP, 1 mile at HMP, 3 miles at MP, 1 mile cool-down, SAM Easy.

W   LMLS, 35-40 minutes easy with 5 x 30 second strides (60-90 seconds easy recovery), SAM Easy.

Th Complete day off from running and cross training.

F   LMLS, 30-35 minutes easy, SAM Easy.

S   Pre-race, 10-15 minute easy running, then 5 x 30 second strides (60-90 seconds easy recovery), then 5-minute cool-down, LS and hip mobility from Phase 1 SAM Easy.

Su Race! Execute a smart race plan and you'll be happy with the result. Remember, be conservative in the opening miles of the race.

SATURDAY RACE TRAINING

Note: SAM Easy for men on Friday; SAM Hard for women on Friday.

WEEK 19

M LMLS, 45 minutes easy with 5 x 30 second strides (60-90 seconds easy recovery), SAM Easy.

T LMLS, 2 miles warm-up, 3 miles at MP, 0.5 miles "fun-fast," 3 miles at MP, 1 mile cool-down, SAM Easy.

W Brisk walk of 45 minutes, LMLS before and SAM Easy afterward is encouraged.

Th LMLS, 35 minutes easy with 5 x 30 second strides (60-90 seconds easy recovery), SAM Easy.

F LMLS, 10 mile long run, 4 miles easy, 5 miles at MP, 1 mile cool-down, SAM immediately after the run (SAM Easy for men, SAM Hard for women).

S Brisk walk of 45 minutes, LMLS before and SAM Easy afterward is encouraged.

Su LMLS, 45 minutes easy with 5 x 30 second strides (60-90 seconds easy recovery), SAM Easy.

WEEK 20

M LMLS, 1 mile warm-up, 2 miles at MP, 1 mile at HMP, 3 miles at MP, 1 mile cool-down, SAM Easy.

T LMLS, 45 minutes easy with 5 x 30 second strides (60-90 seconds easy recovery), SAM Easy.

W Complete day off from running and cross training.

Th LMLS, 35 minutes easy, SAM Easy.

F Pre-race, 10-15 minutes easy running, then 5 x 30 second strides (60-90 seconds easy recovery), then 10 minute cool-down, LS and mobility from SAM Easy.

S Race! Execute a smart race plan and you'll be happy with the result. Remember, be conservative in the opening miles of the race.

Su Start SMT Recovery Phase.

HALF MARATHON TRAINING

— WEEK 1 —

WEEK 1

Note: Just 3 reps of lunges on each side this week for all LMLS warm-ups.

M   LMLS, 45 minutes easy with 5 x 20 second strides (60-90 seconds easy recovery), SAM Easy.

T   LMLS, 10-minute warm-up, 35 minutes of 3 minutes on, 2 minutes steady fartlek, 10-minute cool-down, SAM Hard.

W   LMLS, 50 minutes easy, SAM Easy.

Th LMLS, 45 minutes easy cross training, SAM Easy.

F   LMLS, 40 minutes easy with 5 x 20 second strides (60-90 seconds easy recovery), SAM Easy. Note: Just 3 reps of lunges on each side this week for all LMLS warm-ups.

S   LMLS, 12 miles easy, then immediately into SAM Hard.

Su Brisk walk of 45-60 minutes, LMLS before and SAM Easy afterward is encouraged, but not mandatory.

WEEK 2

Note: Just 4 reps of lunges on each side this week for all LMLS warm-ups.

M   LMLS, 45 minutes easy with 5 x 20 second strides (60-90 seconds easy recovery), SAM Easy.

T   LMLS, 10-minute warm-up, 35 minute progression run: 15 minutes steady, 10 minutes faster, 5 minutes faster, 5 minutes fastest but controlled, 10-minute cool-down, SAM Hard.

W   LMLS, 55 minutes easy, SAM Easy.

Th LMLS, 45-50 minutes easy cross training, SAM Easy.

F   LMLS, 40 minutes easy with 5 x 20 second strides (60-90 seconds easy recovery), SAM Easy.

S   LMLS, 12 miles, if you feel good at the 10 mile mark you can speed up the last two miles, then immediately into SAM Hard.

Su Brisk walk of 45-60 minutes, LMLS before and SAM Easy afterward is encouraged, but not mandatory.

WEEK 3

Note: 5 reps of lunges on each side this week for all LMLS warm-ups. This is the full LM warm-up.

M   LMLS, 50 minutes easy with 5 x 20 second strides (60-90 seconds easy recovery), SAM Easy.

T   LMLS, 10 minute warm-up, 4 x 8 minutes at a challenging pace with 3 minute steady recoveries, 10 minute cool-down, SAM Hard.

W   LMLS, 60 minutes easy, SAM Easy.

Th LMLS, 45-50 minutes easy cross training, SAM Easy.

F   LMLS, 45 minutes easy with 5 x 20 second strides (60-90 seconds easy recovery), SAM Easy.

S   LMLS, 13 miles easy, then immediately into SAM Hard.

Su Brisk walk of 50-65 minutes, LMLS before and SAM Easy afterward is encouraged, but not mandatory.

WEEK 4

M   LMLS, 50 minutes easy with 5 x 20 second strides (60-90 seconds easy recovery), SAM Easy.

T   LMLS, 10-minute warm-up, 20 minutes of 3 minute on, 2 minutes steady, right into 25 minutes of 4 minutes on, 1 minute steady, 10-minute cool-down, SAM Hard.

W   LMLS, 60-65 minutes easy, SAM Easy.

Th LMLS, 45 minutes easy cross training, SAM Easy. Note: Must make sure the cross training is easy today.

F   Pre-race, LMLS, 10-15 minutes easy, 4-5 x 20 second strides (60-90 seconds easy recovery).

S   Pre-race, LMLS, 10-15 minutes easy, 4-5 x 20 second strides, finishing the strides roughly a minute or two before the gun goes off, Execute a great 5k Race! 10 minute cool-down down jog, then SAM Easy after the race.

Su Brisk walk of 35-60 minutes, LMLS before and SAM Easy afterward is encouraged, but not mandatory.

WEEK 5

M	Day off – no running or cross training. If you must do something you can do the mobility work from SAM and you can do rope stretching.
T	LMLS, 60 minutes easy cross training, SAM Easy.
W	LMLS, 45 minutes easy, SAM Hard.
Th	LMLS, 45-55 minutes easy cross training, SAM Easy.
F	LMLS, 45 minutes easy with 5 x 20 second strides (60-90 seconds easy recovery), SAM Easy.
S	LMLS, 14 miles easy, then immediately into SAM Hard.
Su	Brisk walk of 60-75 minutes, LMLS before and SAM Easy afterward is encouraged, but not mandatory.

WEEK 6

M	LMLS, 50 minutes easy with 5 x 25 second strides (60-90 seconds easy recovery), SAM Easy.
T	Pre-race warm-up, Yasso 800s - 8 x 800m with 400m jog, 10 minute cool-down jog, then SAM Hard.
W	LMLS, 60 minutes easy, SAM Easy.
Th	LMLS, 45-60 minutes easy cross training, SAM Easy.
F	LMLS, 45-50 minutes easy with 5 x 25 second strides (60-90 seconds easy recovery), SAM Easy.
S	LMLS, 16 miles easy, then immediately into SAM Hard.
Su	Brisk walk of 60-80 minutes, LMLS before and SAM Easy afterward is encouraged, but not mandatory.

M	LMLS, 55 minutes easy with 5 x 25 second strides (60-90 seconds easy recovery), SAM Easy.
T	LMLS, 10-minute warm-up, 45 minutes of 4 minutes on, 1 minute steady fartlek, 10-minute cool-down, SAM Hard.
W	LMLS, 60-70 minutes easy, SAM Easy.
Th	LMLS, 45-60 minutes easy cross training, SAM Easy.
F	LMLS, 55 minutes easy with 5 x 25 second strides (60-90 seconds easy recovery), SAM Easy.
S	LMLS, 16 miles, if you feel good at the 14 mile mark you can speed up the last 2 miles, then immediately into SAM Hard.
Su	Brisk walk of 60-85 minutes, LMLS before and SAM Easy afterward is encouraged, but not mandatory.

M	LMLS, 55 minutes easy with 5 x 25 second strides (60-90 seconds easy recovery), SAM Easy.
T	LMLS, 10-minute warm-up, 50 minute progressions run: 20 minutes steady, 15 minutes faster, 10 minutes faster, 5 minutes fastest but controlled, 10-minute cool-down, SAM Hard.
W	LMLS, 60-75 minutes easy, SAM Easy.
Th	LMLS, 45-60 minutes easy cross training, SAM Easy.
F	LMLS, 55 minutes easy with 5 x 25 second strides (60-90 seconds easy recovery), SAM Easy.
S	LMLS, 18 miles easy, then immediately into SAM Hard.
Su	Brisk walk of 60-90 minutes, LMLS before and SAM Easy afterward is encouraged, but not mandatory.

Note: 30 sec, not 25 sec, strides.

WEEK 9

M	LMLS, 55 minutes easy with 5 x 30 second strides (60-90 seconds easy recovery), SAM Easy.
T	Pre-race warm-up, Yasso 800s - 9 x 800m with 400m jog, 10 minute cool-down jog, then SAM Hard.
W	LMLS, 60-70 minutes easy, SAM Easy.
Th	LMLS, 45-60 minutes easy cross training, SAM Easy.
F	LMLS, 55 minutes easy with 5 x 30 second strides (60-90 seconds easy recovery), SAM Easy.
S	LMLS, 18 miles, if you feel good at the 15 mile mark you can speed up a bit in the last 3 miles, then immediately into SAM Hard after the run.
Su	Brisk walk of 60-85 minutes, LMLS before and SAM Easy afterward is encouraged, but not mandatory.

WEEK 10

M	LMLS, 55 minutes easy with 5 x 30 second strides (60-90 seconds easy recovery), SAM Easy.
T	LMLS, 10-minute warm-up, 5 x 8 minutes at a challenging pace with 3 minute steady recoveries, 10-minute cool-down, SAM Hard.
W	LMLS, 60-70 minutes easy, SAM Easy.
Th	LMLS, 45-60 minutes easy cross training, SAM Easy.
F	LMLS, 55 minutes easy with 5 x 30 second strides (60-90 seconds easy recovery), SAM Easy.
S	LMLS, 20 miles easy, Just get in the time on your feet, then immediately into SAM Hard after the run.
Su	Brisk walk of 60-85 minutes, LMLS before and SAM Easy afterward is encouraged, but not mandatory.

WEEK 11

M   LMLS, 45 minutes easy with 5 x 30 second strides (60-90 seconds easy recovery), SAM Easy.

T   LMLS, 2 miles warm-up, 3 miles at HMP, 1 mile steady (slower than HMP), 3 miles at HMP, 1 mile cool-down, SAM Hard.

W   LMLS, 60-85 minutes easy, SAM Easy.

Th   LMLS, 45-60 minutes easy cross training, SAM Easy.

F   LMLS, 55 minutes easy with 5 x 30 second strides (60-90 seconds easy recovery), SAM Easy.

S   LMLS, 18 miles, if you feel good at the 14 mile mark you can speed up a bit in the last 4 miles, then immediately into SAM Hard after the run.

Su   Brisk walk of 60-90 minutes, LMLS before and SAM Easy afterward is encouraged, but not mandatory.

WEEK 12

M   LMLS, 55 minutes easy with 5 x 30 second strides (60-90 seconds easy recovery), SAM Easy.

T   LMLS, 2 miles warm-up, 2 miles at HMP, 0.5 miles "fun-fast", 3 miles at HMP, 1 mile cool-down, SAM Hard.

W   LMLS, 60 minutes easy, SAM Easy.

Th   LMLS, 45-60 minutes easy cross training, SAM Easy.

F   LMLS, 45 minutes easy with 5 x 30 second strides (60-90 seconds easy recovery), SAM Easy.

S   LMLS, 12 miles, 6 miles easy, 5 miles at HMP, 1 mile cool-down.

Su   Brisk walk of 45-60 minutes, LMLS before and SAM Easy afterward is encouraged, but not mandatory.

WEEK 13	M	LMLS, 45 minutes easy with 5 x 30 second strides (60-90 seconds easy recovery), SAM Easy.
	T	LMLS, 2 miles warm-up, 2.5 miles at HMP, 0.5 miles "fun-fast", 2 miles at HMP, 1 mile cool-down, SAM Easy.
	W	LMLS, 45 minutes easy with 5 x 30 second strides (60-90 seconds easy recovery), Phase 2 SAM Easy.
	Th	Complete day off from running and cross training.
	F	LMLS, 35 minute easy run, Phase 1 SAM Easy.
	S	Pre-race, LMLS, 10-15 minute warm-up, 5 x 30 second strides (60-90 seconds easy recovery), 5-minute cool-down, hip mobility from Phase 1 SAM Easy.
	Su	Race Half Marathon! Pre-race routine, race, then LS after the race then hip mobility from Phase 1 SAM Easy at night.

WEEK 14	M	30 minute easy jog/walk to do a body scan and see what is sore and needs attention in the coming days. Hip mobility from Phase 2 SAM Easy and rope stretching.
	T	Brisk walk for 30-60 minutes.
	W	Off, Hip mobility from Phase 2 SAM Easy and rope stretching.
	Th	Cross train for 45 minutes, Go very easy.
	F	Off, hip mobility from Phase 2 SAM Easy and rope stretching.
	S	LMLS, 30-45 minutes easy, SAM Easy.
	Su	Brisk walk for 30-60 minutes.

WEEK 15

M   LMLS, 35 minutes easy with 5 x 30 second strides (60-90 seconds easy recovery), SAM Easy.

T   LMLS, 45 minutes easy with 5 x 30 second strides (60-90 seconds easy recovery), SAM Easy.

W   LMLS, 30 minutes easy run with SAM Easy and rope stretching.

Th LMLS, 45-60 minutes easy cross training, SAM Easy.

F   LMLS, 35 minutes easy with 5 x 30 second strides (60-90 seconds easy recovery), Phase 2 SAM Easy.

S   LM, 20 mile easy run, then immediately into SAM Hard after the run.

Su Brisk walk of 60-90 minutes, LMLS before and SAM Easy afterward is encouraged, but not mandatory.

WEEK 16

M   LMLS, 50 minutes easy with 5 x 30 second strides (60-90 seconds easy recovery), SAM Easy.

T   LMLS, 10-minute warm-up, 40 minute at MP then 5 minutes "fun-fast," finishing with 15 minutes at MP, 10-minute cool-down, SAM Hard.

W   LMLS, 60-70 minutes easy, SAM Easy.

Th LMLS, 35-50 minutes easy cross training, SAM Easy.

F   LMLS, 40 minutes easy with 5 x 30 second strides (60-90 seconds easy recovery), SAM Easy.

S   LMLS, 22 miles, The longest run of the training cycle, Run the first 10 miles conservatively, SAM Easy (not SAM Hard) immediately after the run.

Su Brisk walk of 60-90 minutes, LMLS before and SAM Easy afterward is encouraged, but not mandatory, if you have time, 20-30 minutes of easy walking in the evening is encouraged.

WEEK 17

M	Complete day off from running and cross training.
T	LMLS, 45 minutes easy with 5 x 30 second strides (60-90 seconds easy recovery), SAM Easy.
W	LMLS, 60-70 minutes easy, SAM Easy.
Th	LMLS, 45-60 minutes easy cross training, SAM Easy.
F	LMLS, 50 minutes easy with 5 x 30 second strides (60-90 seconds easy recovery), SAM Easy.
S	LMLS, 16 mile long run, 7 miles easy, 8 miles at MP, 1 mile cool-down, then immediately into SAM Hard after the run.
Su	Brisk walk of 60-90 minutes, LMLS before and SAM Easy afterward is encouraged, but not mandatory.

WEEK 18

M	LMLS, 55 minutes easy with 5 x 30 second strides (60-90 seconds easy recovery), SAM Easy.
T	LMLS, 2 miles warm-up, 4 miles at MP, 1 mile at HMP, 3 miles at MP, 1 mile cool-down, SAM Hard.
W	LMLS, 60-70 minutes easy, SAM Easy.
Th	LMLS, 45-60 minutes easy cross training, SAM Easy.
F	LMLS, 45-50 minutes easy with 5 x 30 second strides (60-90 seconds easy recovery), SAM Easy.
S	LMLS, 14 mile long run, 6 miles easy, 7 miles at MP, 1 mile cool-down, then immediately into SAM Hard after the run.
Su	Brisk walk of 60 minutes, LMLS before and SAM Easy afterward is encouraged, but not mandatory.

M   LMLS, 50 minutes easy with 5 x 30 second strides (60-90 seconds easy recovery), SAM Easy.

T   LMLS, 2 miles warm-up, 3 miles at MP, 0.5 miles "fun-fast," 3 miles at MP, 1 mile cool-down, SAM Hard.

W   LMLS, 60-minute easy run, SAM Easy.

Th   LMLS, 45 minutes easy cross training, SAM Easy.

F   LMLS, 45 minutes easy with 5 x 30 second strides (60-90 seconds easy recovery), SAM Easy.

S   LMLS, 12 mile long run, 5 miles easy, 6 miles at MP, 1 mile cool-down, SAM immediately after the run, SAM Hard for women, SAM Easy for men.

Su   Brisk walk of 45 minutes, LMLS before and SAM Easy afterward is encouraged, but not

M   LMLS, 40 minutes easy with 5 x 30 second strides (60-90 seconds easy recovery), SAM Easy.

T   LMLS, 1 mile warm-up, 2 miles at MP, 1 mile at HMP, 3 miles at MP, 1 mile cool-down, SAM Easy.

W   LMLS, 35-40 minutes with 5 x 30 second strides (60-90 seconds easy recovery), SAM Easy.

Th   Complete day off from running and cross training.

F   LMLS, 30-35 minute easy run, SAM Easy.

S   Pre-race, 10-15 minutes of easy running, then 5 x 30 second strides (60-90 seconds easy recovery), then 10 minutes cool-down, LS and hip mobility from Phase 1 SAM Easy.

Su   Race! Execute a smart race plan and you'll be happy with the result, Be conservative in the opening miles of the race.

8 WEEKS TO SMT TRAINING

WEEK 1

Note: LM: Three Lunges per leg, per exercise

M	LMLS, 20-25 minute easy run, SAM Easy.
T	LMLS, 30-35 minute easy run, SAM Easy.
W	Brisk 45 minute walk.
Th	Off.
F	LMLS, 20-25 minute easy run, SAM Easy.
S	LMLS, 3 miles easy, SAM Easy.
Su	Brisk 45 minute walk.

WEEK 2

M	LMLS, 25 minute easy run, SAM Easy.
T	LMLS, 30-35 minute easy run, SAM Easy.
W	Brisk 45 minute walk.
Th	Off.
F	LMLS, 25 minute easy run, SAM Easy.
S	LMLS, 4 miles easy, SAM Easy.
Su	Brisk 45 minute walk.

WEEK 3

Note: LM: Four Lunges per leg, per exercise

M   LMLS, 30 minute easy run, SAM Easy.

T   LMLS, 40 minute easy run, SAM Easy.

W   Brisk 45 minute walk.

Th   Off.

F   LMLS, 30 minute easy run, SAM Easy.

S   LMLS, 5 miles easy, SAM Easy.

Su   Brisk 45 minute walk.

WEEK 4

M   LMLS, 35-40 minute easy run, SAM Easy.

T   LMLS, 40-45 minute easy run, SAM Easy.

W   Brisk 45 minute walk.

Th   Off.

F   LMLS, 35 minute easy run, SAM Easy.

S   LMLS, 6 miles easy, SAM Easy.

Su   Brisk 55-65 minute walk.

WEEK 5

Note: LM: Five Lunges per leg, per exercise

M   LMLS, 40 minute easy run, SAM Easy.

T   LMLS, 45 minute easy run, SAM Easy.

W   Brisk 50 minute walk.

Th   Off.

F   LMLS, 35 minute easy run, SAM Easy.

S   LMLS, 6-7 miles easy, SAM Easy.

Su   Brisk 55-65 minute walk.

WEEK 6

M	LMLS, 45 minute easy run, SAM Easy.
T	LMLS, 50 minutes easy run, SAM Easy.
W	Brisk 50 minute walk.
Th	Off.
F	LMLS, 40 minute easy run, SAM Easy.
S	LMLS, 7 miles easy, SAM Easy.
Su	Brisk 60-75 minute walk.

WEEK 7

M	LMLS, 45 minute easy run, SAM Easy.
T	LMLS, 50-55 minute easy run, SAM Easy.
W	Brisk 55 minute walk.
Th	Off.
F	LMLS, 40-45 minute easy run, SAM Easy.
S	LMLS, 8 miles easy, SAM Easy.
Su	Brisk 60-75 minute walk.

WEEK 8

M	LMLS, 45 minute easy run, SAM Easy.
T	LMLS, 55 minute easy run, SAM Easy.
W	Brisk 55 minute walk.
Th	Off.
F	LMLS, 30 minute easy run, SAM Easy.
S	LMLS, 9 miles easy, SAM Easy.
Su	Brisk 45 minute walk.

APPENDIX

"There is no real ending. It's just the place where you stop the story."

— Frank Herbert

SEMI-PERSONAL COACHING

The Simple Marathon Training system is indeed simple, and for most readers it is the perfect guide to be prepared to run a great marathon. I also offer Semi-Personal Coaching that follows the SMT system, giving you more guidance and personalized specifics to help you along the path to race day. Semi-Personal Coaching from *SimpleMarathonTraining.com* is comprised of four elements. First, a video delivered each week that summarizes the week's training. Second, a daily email during both the 20-week training cycle and the 4-week recovery cycle to ensure that you know what to do each and every day. Third, guided audio workouts for the first three Tuesday workouts of the 20-week cycle, which will help you learn to run by feel. Fourth, access to a forum where you can ask me questions about training and how to adjust the SMT system for your individual life. While I can't guarantee that I will be able to answer every question, this is a unique opportunity for you and me to interact and make sure you are getting the most out of the SMT system. Visit *SimpleMarathonTraining.com* for more information.

I would love to hear about your journey during the 20-week training cycle. Find me and other trainees on:

facebook.com/SimpleMarathonTraining
pinterest.com/SimpleRunning
instagram/SimpleRunningTraining
@SimpleMarathon on twitter

Get in touch with your fellow marathoners by using the following hashtags when you post about a workout or race:

#simplemarathontraining #SMT #simplemarathon
#simplemarathonrunning #simplerunningtraining #SRT
#simplerunning #whenindoubtdoless #WIDDL #simpleainteasy
#SAM #knockedoutSAM #strengthandmobility #strongchassis
#marathonpace #loveMPworkouts #grooveMP #fartlek
#progressionrun #tiredlegswednesday #easyrunandstrides
#ERAS (easy run and strides) #easydayseasy #22milelongrun
#20milelongrun #18milelongrun #trainsmartracefast #SMTMoms
#MarathonMoms #MomsloveSAM #Semipersonalcoaching

GLOSSARY

Fartlek   Swedish term that means "speed-play." Fartlek workouts have alternating paces, most commonly between two paces. While paces can be assigned for fartlek workouts, in the SMT system the fartlek running is done by feel, with no specified pace for the "on" and "steady" portion. The "steady" pace should be run faster than easy pace, while the "on" should be yet another jump in pace. The most common mistake with a fartlek workout is to run the "on" portion too fast and the "steady" portion too slowly. Incorrectly running a fartlek workout the first couple of times is a great tool for learning to run by feel.

Fun Fast   Fun Fast is a pace that is faster than marathon pace (MP) and is used in MP workouts to both create a more demanding aerobic workout and to get the runner out of MP biomechanics and into slightly different mechanics (e.g., higher knee lift). Fun Fast is a subjective term, but by the time Fun Fast is employed in the SMT system, runners will have an intuitive sense of the pace. More concretely, Fun Fast is a pace a runner could run for a 5k race. The key with Fun Fast running in the SMT system is that it is challenging, yet controlled running.

Half-Marathon Pace (HMP)   In the SMT system, half marathon pace is the pace calculated with an online calculator based on the Yasso 800s workout. Half marathon pace is a guide for workouts in the SMT system where there is alteration between marathon pace (MP) and half marathon pace (HMP).

Leg Swings (LS)   Leg Swings prepare the hip joint for the demands of running in two ways: 1. Challenging the range of motion and 2. Pumping synovial fluid into the hip joint (via imbibition).

LMLS   Short for Lunge Matrix and Leg Swings. In the SMT system runners go through the LMLS routine before every run and cross training workout. The routine requires approximately five minutes to complete.

Lunge Matrix (LM)   The Lunge Matrix used in the SMT system is rooted in the work of Dr. Gary Gray. The lunge matrix consists of five lunges: front lunge, front lunge with twist, side lunge, back lunge, to the side lunge, and backwards lunge. Athletes work up to doing five reps of each lunge on each side, for a total of 50 lunges. The lunge matrix is a powerful warm-up tool for runners because it forces the runner to move in all three planes of motion. Running is primarily a sagittal plane activity (with a slight amount of transverse plane movement at the shoulders and hips). The LM helps prepare the body for the demands of running.

Marathon Pace (MP)   Marathon pace is the pace that you hope to run on race day. In other training programs this would be referred to as goal pace. There is MP in every week of the final six weeks of SMT.

SAM   SAM is short for Strength And Mobility, specifically core strength, hip strength, and hip mobility. These three aspects are fundamental to the SMT system and SMT runners will do some sort of SAM work after every run. SAM is organized by phases, starting with Phase 1, and categorized into SAM Easy and SAM Hard. After a running workout, the runner will immediately start SAM, maintaining the elevated heart rate and thereby lengthening the aerobic stimulus of the workout.

SAM Easy   SAM Easy days follow the running portions of Monday, Wednesday, and Friday, as well as the Thursday cross-training day.

SAM Hard   SAM Hard days follow the Tuesday workout and the Saturday long run.

Strides   In the SMT system a stride is 20-30 seconds at 5k pace with 60-90 seconds of easy jogging as recovery. Strides are part of Monday and Friday, as well as part of the pre-race work done the day before a race. In the SMT system, strides are done within the run, not after the run, as is the case in most training plans. Doing the strides in the middle of the run saves the runner time and helps the runner (on most occasions) feel strong and energetic at the end of the run. Note: if the goal of training is to run a 5k race, then the strides would start at 5k pace and gradually increase.

Taper   The goal of a taper is to prepare an athlete to perform their best in their goal competition. A taper is a significant decrease in volume, coupled with a slight decrease in intensity. In the SMT system the last three weeks of the 20-week training cycle can be considered a taper as the volume of running decreases, yet the percentage of running done at marathon pace or faster is significant.

Volume   The number of minutes, miles, or kilometers a runner completes in a given day, week, or training cycle.

Yasso 800s   Bart Yasso is the creator of this workout, which is both a challenging workout and a predictor of marathon performance. The workout is 8-10 x 800m, with a 400m recovery in the same time it takes to run the 800m segment. For instance, if a runner runs 3 minutes and 30 seconds for the 800m, the 400m rest lap is 3 minutes and 30 seconds. The predictive aspect of the workout is as follows: the average minutes and seconds of the 800m correspond to the hours and minutes it would take them to run the marathon, respectively. A runner who runs three minutes and thirty seconds for the 800m repeats can project a 3 hours and 30 minutes marathon time. However, most runners find that they need to add 5 minutes to their predicted marathon time. In the previous example, the runner should expect a goal marathon time of 3 hours and 35 minutes based on 3:30 Yasso 800m pace. Yasso 800s have a significant place in the SMT system, the workout is employed three times in the 20-week cycle.

———— RESOURCES ————

Performance Calculators

The calculator at *www.mcmillanrunning.com* is far and away the most popular calculator. I use it often and it's a great tool. However, you need to understand the calculator's limitations. The first limitation is that the calculator is most accurate for a distance just shorter or just longer of the distance being used in the calculator. When you put in your latest 10k performance, the prediction for the 5k and the half marathon are reasonably accurate, but projecting for a marathon becomes problematic. Further, the problem with thinking you can run the 5k and half marathon time that the calculator spits out is that you would have to do some race pace work—specificity at 5k pace or half marathon pace—to run the performance that the calculator projects. For the half marathon, you will also need to be running more volume than a 10k requires. The final point to be made is that the SMT system uses the calculator to predict a marathon performance based on the 5k run in Week 4 of the training. You should be able to run the predicted marathon if you get in all of the training in the SMT system between the 5k in Week 4 and the marathon in Week 20.

Books

Run: The Mind-Body Method of Running by Feel by Matt Fitzgerald

This book does a great job of explaining how to run by feel and how many of the best runners in the world employ running by feel to reach their potential as athletes. Fitzgerald's writing is clear and concise, and Matt is a consummate student of the sport. A runner who follows the SMT system will come to understand the importance of running by feel, and this book supports the important role of running by feel in intelligent training programs.

The Science of Running: How to Find your Limit and Train to Maximize your Performance by Steve Magness

Just as the title suggests, this book is rooted in scientific studies and is only for the runner who wants to dive deep into the minutiae of exercise physiology and how it relates to running. If you like the Geek Out sections by Dr. Carwyn Sharp and Dr. Trent Stellingwerff, you will find this book very informative. What I like about the book is that Steve has coached high school, collegiate, and professional athletes and has taken theories in exercise physiology and applied them to help his athletes run faster.

Advanced Marathoning (2nd Edition) by Pete Pfitzinger and Scott Douglas

I've included this book for several reasons, the first of which is that Pfitzinger and Douglas are two of the most knowledgeable people in marathon training. Pfitzinger is a former world-class marathoner and exercise physiologist, and Douglas is a seasoned writer, editor, and author. Thousands of runners have run PRs in the marathon using this book, and it has indeed become the measure of a marathon training book. The SMT system is designed for busy adults with hectic lives; if you have enough time in your life to follow the training laid out in *Advanced Marathoning* you will be well served not only in training, but also on race day. If this is the resource you choose to use because your schedule allows for it, I would highly recommend supplementing the training with SAM.

A Cold Clear Day by Frank Murphy

This is the story of Buddy Edelen, an American marathon runner who raced in the early 1960s under the guidance of coach Fred Wilt. In our current age of digital communication through phones and computers, it's extremely interesting to follow the coach-athlete relationship done through letters with a lag time of several weeks. This is a quick read that you'll enjoy reading for a second or third time.

Once a Runner by John L. Parker, Jr.

Parker's novel has become a classic because of the pitch perfect voice that conveys the experience and intangible spirit of what it is to be a competitive runner. The star of the book, Quenton Cassidy, pursues the dream of being a champion miler, and the reader is with him every step of the way.

275

GEEK OUT
REFERENCES

Carwyn Sharp PhD – Your Long Run

(Note: A number of historical research papers have been used to highlight how long this knowledge has been around and to give credit to the early exercise science pioneers upon whose shoulders we now stand as scientists, coaches and athletes. This work has been verified countless times in the decades since.)

1. Jentjens, R., and Jeukendrup, A. E. (2003). Determinants of post-exercise glycogen synthesis during short-term recovery. Sports Medicine, 33(2), 117-144.
2. Holloszy, J.O., and E.F. Coyle (1984). Adaptations of skeletal muscle to endurance exercise and their metabolic consequences. J. Appl. Physiol. 56: 831-838.
3. Karlsson, J., L.O. Nordesjo, L. Jorfeldt, and B. Saltin (1972). Muscle lactate, ATP, and CP levels during exercise after physical training in man. J. Appl. Physiol. 33: 199-203.
4. Holloszy, J.O. (1967). Biochemical adaptations in muscle. Effects of exercise on mitochondrial oxygen uptake and respiratory enzyme activity in skeletal muscle. J. Biol. Chem. 242: 2278-2282.
5. Booth, F.W. (1977). Effects of endurance exercise on cytochrome c turnover in skeletal muscle. Annals N. Y. Acad. Sci. 301: 431-439.
6. Holloszy, J.O. (1967). Biochemical adaptations in muscle. Effects of exercise on mitochondrial oxygen uptake and respiratory enzyme activity in skeletal muscle. J. Biol. Chem. 242: 2278-2282.
7. Pette, D., and Staron, R. S. (2000). Myosin isoforms, muscle fiber types, and transitions. Microscopy research and technique, 50(6), 500-509.
8. Sawka, M. N., Convertino, V. A., Eichner, E. R., Schnieder, S. M., & Young, A. J. (2000). Blood volume: importance and adaptations to exercise training, environmental stresses, and trauma/sickness. Medicine and science in sports and exercise, 32(2), 332-348.
9. Swank, A. and Sharp, C. (2015). Adaptations to Aerobic Endurance Training Programs, In G.G. Haff and N.T. Triplett (Eds.), Essentials of Strength Training and Conditioning (pp. 115-133). Champaign, IL: Human Kinetics.
10. Blomqvist, C. G., and Saltin, B. (1983). Cardiovascular adaptations to physical training. Annual Review of Physiology, 45(1), 169-189.
11. Dudley, G.A., W.M. Abraham, and R.L. Terjung (1982). Influence of exercise intensity and duration on biochemical adaptations in skeletal muscle. J. Appl. Physiol. 53: 844-850.
12. Hawley, J. A. (2002). Adaptations of skeletal muscle to prolonged, intense

endurance training. Clinical and experimental pharmacology and physiology, 29(3), 218-222.

Carwyn Sharp PhD – Concurrent Training and Endurance Training

1. Tipton, KD, and Wolfe, RR. Exercise-induced changes in protein metabolism. Acta Physiol Scand 162:377-387, 1998.
2. Silverman, HG, and Mazzeo, RS. Hormonal responses to maximal and submaximal exercise in trained and untrained men of various ages. J Gerontol A Biol Sci Med Sci 51:B30-B37, 1996.
3. Tuna, Z, Güzel, NA, Aral, AL, Elbeg, S, Özer, C, Erikoglu, G, Atak, A, and Pinar, L. Effects of an acute exercise up to anaerobic threshold on serum anabolic and catabolic factors in trained and sedentary young males. Gazi Med J 25:47-51, 2014.
4. Trappe, S, Harber, M, Creer, A, Gallagher, P, Slivka, D, Minchev, K, and Whitsett, D. Single muscle fiber adaptations with marathon training. J Appl Physiol 101:721-727, 2006.
5. Wilkinson, SB, Phillips, SM, Atherton, PJ, Patel, R, Yarasheski, KE, Tarnopolsky, MA, and Rennie, MJ. Differential effects of resistance and endurance exercise in the fed state on signalling molecule phosphorylation and protein synthesis in human muscle. J Physiol, 586:3701-3717, 2008.
6. MacDougall JD, Sale DG, Moroz JR, Elder GC, Sutton JR, Howald H. Mitochondrial volume density in human skeletal muscle following heavy resistance training. Med Sci Sports. 1979;11(2):164-6.
7. Hennessy LC, & Watson AWS. The interference effects of training for strength and endurance simultaneously. 1994 15:326-31.
8. McCarthy, J. P., Agre, J. C., Graf, B. K., Pozniak, M. A., & Vailas, A. C. (1995). Compatibility of adaptive responses with combining strength and endurance training. Medicine and science in sports and exercise, 27(3), 429-436.
9. Hickson RC, Rosenkoetter MA, & Brown MM. Strength training effects on aerobic power and short-term endurance. Med Sci Sports Exerc. 1980;12(5):336-9
10. Hickson RC, Dvorak BA, Gorostiaga EM, Kurowski TT, & Foster C. Potential for strength and endurance training to amplify endurance performance. J Appl Physiol. 1988;65(5):2285-90.
11. Marcinik EJ, Potts J, Schlabach G, Will S, Dawson P, & Hurley BF. Effects of strength training on lactate threshold and endurance performance. Med Sci Sports Exerc. 1991;23(6):739-43.
12. Chilibeck PD, Syrotuik DG, & Bell GJ. The effect of concurrent endurance and strength training on quantitative estimates of subsarcolemmal and intermyofibrillar mitochondria. Int J Sports Med. 2002;23(1):33-9.
13. Yamamoto, L. M., Lopez, R. M., Klau, J. F., Casa, D. J., Kraemer, W. J., & Maresh, C. M. (2008). The effects of resistance training on endurance distance running performance among highly trained runners: a systematic review. The Journal of Strength & Conditioning Research, 22(6), 2036-2044.
14. Sedano, S, Marin, PJ, Cuadrado, G, and Redondo, JC. Concurrent training in elite male runners: The influence of strength versus muscular endurance training on performance outcomes. J Strength Cond Res 27:2433-2443, 2013.
15. Dudley, GA, and Djamil, R. Incompatibility of endurance- and strength-training modes of exercise. J Appl Physiol 59:1446-1451, 1985.

16. Bell, GJ, Syrotuik, D, Martin, TP, Burnham, R, and Quinney, HA. Effect of concurrent strength and endurance training on skeletal muscle properties and hormone concentrations in humans. Eur J Appl Physiol 81:418-427, 2000.

17. McCarthy, J. P., Agre, J. C., Graf, B. K., Pozniak, M. A., & Vailas, A. C. (1995). Compatibility of adaptive responses with combining strength and endurance training. Medicine and science in sports and exercise, 27(3), 429-436.

18. McCarthy, JP, Pozniak, MA, and Agre, JC. Neuromuscular adaptations to concurrent strength and endurance training. Med Sci Sports Exerc 34:511-519, 2002.

19. Leveritt, M, Abernethy, PJ, Barry, B, and Logan, PA. Concurrent strength and endurance training: The influence of dependent variable selection. J Strength Cond Res 17:503-508, 2003.

20. Paavolainen L, Hakkinen K, Hamalainen I, Nummela A, & Rusko H. Explosive-strength training improves 5-km running time by improving running economy and muscle power. J Appl Physiol. 1999;86(5):1527-33.

21. Skoluda, N, Dettenborn, L, Stalder, T, and Kirschbaum, C. Elevated hair cortisol concentrations in endurance athletes. Psychoneuroendocrinology 37:611-617, 2012

22. Wilson, JM, Marin, PJ, Rhea, MR, Wilson, SM, Loenneke, JP, and Anderson, JC. Concurrent training: A meta-analysis examining interference of aerobic and resistance exercises. J Strength Cond Res 26:2293-2307, 2012.

Carwyn Sharp PhD – The Latest Sleep Science

1. Hublin, C., Kaprio, J., Partinen, M., & Koskenvuo, M. (2001). Insufficient sleep-a population-based study in adults. Sleep, 24(4), 392-400.

2. Lastella, M., Roach, G. D., Halson, S. L., & Sargent, C. (2015). Sleep/wake behaviours of elite athletes from individual and team sports. European journal of sport science, 15(2), 94-100.

3. Morris, C. J., Aeschbach, D., & Scheer, F. A. (2012). Circadian system, sleep and endocrinology. Molecular and cellular endocrinology, 349(1), 91-104.

4. Radogna, F., Diederich, M. & Ghibelli, L. (2010). Melatonin: a pleiotropic molecule regulating inflammation. Biochemical pharmacology, 80(12), 1844-1852.

5. Reiter, R. J., Calvo, J. R., Karbownik, M., Qi, W., & Tan, D. X. (2000). Melatonin and its relation to the immune system and inflammation. Annals of the New York Academy of Sciences, 917(1), 376-386.

6. Morris, C. J., Aeschbach, D., & Scheer, F. A. (2012). Circadian system, sleep and endocrinology. Molecular and cellular endocrinology, 349(1), 91-104.

7. Goel, N., Rao, H., Durmer, J. S., & Dinges, D. F. (2009, September). Neurocognitive consequences of sleep deprivation. In Seminars in neurology (Vol. 29, No. 4, p. 320). NIH Public Access.

8. AlDabal, L., & BaHammam, A. S. (2011). Metabolic, endocrine, and immune consequences of sleep deprivation. Open Respir Med J, 5(1), 31-43.

9. Greer, S. M., Goldstein, A. N., & Walker, M. P. (2013). The impact of sleep deprivation on food desire in the human brain. Nature communications, 4.

10. Halson, S. L. (2008). Nutrition, sleep and recovery. European Journal of sport science, 8(2), 119-126.

11. Milewski, M. D., Skaggs, D. L., Bishop, G. A., Pace, J. L., Ibrahim, D. A., Wren,

T. A., & Barzdukas, A. (2014). Chronic lack of sleep is associated with increased sports injuries in adolescent athletes. Journal of Pediatric Orthopaedics, 34(2), 129-133.

12. Halson, S. L., Martin, D. T., Gardner, A. S., Fallon, K., & Gulbin, J. (2006). Persistent fatigue in a female sprint cyclist after a talent transfer initiative. International Journal of Sports Physiology and Performance, 1, 65-69.

13. Maquet, P. (2001). The role of sleep in learning and memory. Science, 294(5544), 1048-1052.

14. Reilly, T., & Edwards, B. (2007). Altered sleep wake cycles and physical performance in athletes. Physiology and Behavior, 90, 274-284.

15. Goel, N., Rao, H., Durmer, J. S., & Dinges, D. F. (2009, September). Neurocognitive consequences of sleep deprivation. In Seminars in neurology (Vol. 29, No. 4, p. 320). NIH Public Access.

16. Van Dongen, H. P., Vitellaro, K. M., & Dinges, D. F. (2005). Individual differences in adult human sleep and wakefulness: Leitmotif for a research agenda. Sleep, 28(4), 479-496.

17. Goel, N., Rao, H., Durmer, J. S., & Dinges, D. F. (2009, September). Neurocognitive consequences of sleep deprivation. In Seminars in neurology (Vol. 29, No. 4, p. 320). NIH Public Access.

18. Epstein, L.J., & M. Steven (Eds). (2008) The Harvard Medical School Guide to a Good Night's Sleep. The McGraw-Hill Companies: New York, NY.

19. Mah, C. Extended Sleep and the Effects on Mood and Athletic Performance in Collegiate Swimmers. Annual Meeting of the Associated Professional Sleep Societies. June 9, 2008.

20. Mah, C. D., Mah, K. E., Kezirian, E. J., & Dement, W. C. (2011). The effects of sleep extension on the athletic performance of collegiate basketball players. Sleep, 34(7), 943.

21. Halson, S. L., Martin, D. T., Gardner, A. S., Fallon, K., & Gulbin, J. (2006). Persistent fatigue in a female sprint cyclist after a talent transfer initiative. International Journal of Sports Physiology and Performance, 1, 65-69.

22. Halson, S. L. (2008). Nutrition, sleep and recovery. European Journal of sport science, 8(2), 119-126

23. Halson, S. L. (2008). Nutrition, sleep and recovery. European Journal of sport science, 8(2), 119-126.

24. Waterhouse, J., Atkinson, G., Edwards, B., & Reilly, T. (2007). The role of a short post-lunch nap in improving cognitive, motor, and sprint performance in participants with partial sleep deprivation. Journal of sports sciences, 25(14), 1557-1566.

25. Hayashi, M., Masuda, A., & Hori, T. (2003). The alerting effects of caffeine, bright light and face washing after a short daytime nap. Clinical neurophysiology, 114(12), 2268-2278.

26. Caffeine Informer. http://www.caffeineinformer.com/the-15-top-energy-drink-brands Accessed April 9th, 2016.

27. E-Imports: Espresso Business Solutions. http://www.e-importz.com/coffee-statistics.php Accessed April 9th, 2016.

28. Harvard Medical School: Harvard Medical Publications (2007) http://www.health.harvard.edu/staying-healthy/repaying-your-sleep-debt. Revised August 2007. Accessed April 9th, 2016

29. (AlDabal and BaHammam, 2011; Greer, et. al., 2013; Halson, 2008; Milewski, et. al., 2014)

Carwyn Sharp PhD – Caffeine Long Run

1. Pedersen, D. J., Lessard, S. J., Coffey, V. G., Churchley, E. G., Wootton, A. M., Watt, M. J., & Hawley, J. A. (2008). High rates of muscle glycogen resynthesis after exhaustive exercise when carbohydrate is coingested with caffeine. Journal of Applied Physiology, 105(1), 7-13.

Carwyn Sharp PhD – Delayed Onset Muscle Soreness (DOMS)

1. Lemon PW, Tarnopolsky MA, MacDougall JD, Atkinson SA. Protein requirements and muscle mass/strength changes during intensive training in novice bodybuilders. J Appl Physiol 1992;73:767.
2. Armstrong, R. B. (1984). Mechanisms of exercise-induced delayed onset muscular soreness: a brief review. Medicine and science in sports and exercise, 16(6), 529-538.
3. Talag, T. S. (1973). Residual muscular soreness as influenced by concentric, eccentric, and static contractions. Research Quarterly. American Association for Health, Physical Education and Recreation, 44(4), 458-469.
4. Armstrong, R. B. (1986). Muscle damage and endurance events. Sports medicine, 3(5), 370-381.
5. Braun, W. A., & Dutto, D. J. (2003). The effects of a single bout of downhill running and ensuing delayed onset of muscle soreness on running economy performed 48 h later. European journal of applied physiology, 90(1-2), 29-34.
6. Warren, G. L., Ingalls, C. P., Lowe, D. A., & Armstrong, R. B. (2001). Excitation-contraction uncoupling: major role in contraction-induced muscle injury. Exercise and sport sciences reviews, 29(2), 82-87.
7. Rowlands, A. V., Eston, R. G., & Tilzey, C. (2001). Effect of stride length manipulation on symptoms of exercise-induced muscle damage and the repeated bout effect. Journal of sports sciences, 19(5), 333-340.
8. Lemon PW, Tarnopolsky MA, MacDougall JD, Atkinson SA. Protein requirements and muscle mass/strength changes during intensive training in novice bodybuilders. J Appl Physiol 1992;73:767.
9. Ebbeling, C. B., & Clarkson, P. M. (1989). Exercise-induced muscle damage and adaptation. Sports Medicine, 7(4), 207-234.
10. Howatson, G., & Van Someren, K. A. (2008). The prevention and treatment of exercise-induced muscle damage. Sports Medicine, 38(6), 483-503.
11. Howarth, K. R., Moreau, N. A., Phillips, S. M., & Gibala, M. J. (2009). Coingestion of protein with carbohydrate during recovery from endurance exercise stimulates skeletal muscle protein synthesis in humans. Journal of Applied Physiology, 106(4), 1394-1402.
12. Etheridge, T., Philp, A., & Watt, P. W. (2008). A single protein meal increases recovery of muscle function following an acute eccentric exercise bout. Applied physiology, nutrition, and metabolism, 33(3), 483-488.
13. Maridakis, V., O'Connor, P. J., Dudley, G. A., & McCully, K. K. (2007). Caffeine attenuates delayed-onset muscle pain and force loss following eccentric exercise. The Journal of Pain, 8(3), 237-243.
14. Cheung, K., Hume, P. A., & Maxwell, L. (2003). Delayed onset muscle soreness. Sports Medicine, 33(2), 145-164.
15. Tufano, J. J., Brown, L. E., Coburn, J. W., Tsang, K. K., Cazas, V. L., & LaPorta,

J. W. (2012). Effect of aerobic recovery intensity on delayed-onset muscle soreness and strength. The Journal of Strength & Conditioning Research, 26(10), 2777-2782.

16. Peterson, J. M., Trappe, T. A., Mylona, E. L. E. N. I., White, F. A. B. E. R., Lambert, C. P., Evans, W. J., & Pizza, F. X. (2003). Ibuprofen and acetaminophen: effect on muscle inflammation after eccentric exercise. Medicine and science in sports and exercise, 35(6), 892-896.

17. Trappe, T. A., White, F., Lambert, C. P., Cesar, D., Hellerstein, M., & Evans, W. J. (2002). Effect of ibuprofen and acetaminophen on postexercise muscle protein synthesis. American Journal of Physiology-Endocrinology and Metabolism, 282(3), E551-E556.

18. Kraemer, W. J., Bush, J. A., Wickham, R. B., Denegar, C. R., Gómez, A. L., Gotshalk, L. A., ... & Sebastianelli, W. J. (2001). Influence of compression therapy on symptoms following soft tissue injury from maximal eccentric exercise. Journal of Orthopaedic & Sports Physical Therapy, 31(6), 282-290.

19. Davies, V., Thompson, K. G., & Cooper, S. M. (2009). The effects of compression garments on recovery. The Journal of Strength & Conditioning Research, 23(6), 1786-1794.

Trent Stellingwerff PhD – The Science of Optimizing Fueling During the Marathon

1. Stellingwerff T, Boon H, Gijsen AP, Stegen JH, Kuipers H, van Loon LJ: Carbohydrate supplementation during prolonged cycling exercise spares muscle glycogen but does not affect intramyocellular lipid use. Pflügers Archiv : European journal of physiology 2007, 454:635-647.

2. Jeukendrup: Carbohydrate and exercise performance: the role of multiple transportable carbohydrates. Current opinion in clinical nutrition and metabolic care 2010, 13:452-457.

3. Stellingwerff T, Cox GR: Systematic review: Carbohydrate supplementation on exercise performance or capacity of varying durations. Appl Physiol Nutr Metab 2014, 39:998-1011.

4. Pfeiffer B, Stellingwerff T, Hodgson AB, Randell R, Pottgen K, Res P, Jeukendrup AE: Nutritional intake and gastrointestinal problems during competitive endurance events. Medicine and science in sports and exercise 2012, 44:344-351.

5. Stellingwerff T: Case study: nutrition and training periodization in three elite marathon runners. International journal of sport nutrition and exercise metabolism 2012, 22:392-400.

Trent Stellingwerff PhD – The Science of Heat Acclimation

1. Racinais S, Alonso JM, Coutts AJ, Flouris AD, Girard O, Gonzalez-Alonso J, Hausswirth C, Jay O, Lee JK, Mitchell N, et al: Consensus Recommendations on Training and Competing in the Heat. Sports Med 2015, 45:925-938.

2. Garrett AT, Creasy R, Rehrer NJ, Patterson MJ, Cotter JD: Effectiveness of short-term heat acclimation for highly trained athletes. European Journal of

Applied Physiology 2012, 112:1827-1837.
3. Lorenzo S, Halliwill JR, Sawka MN, Minson CT: Heat acclimation improves exercise performance. Journal of Applied Physiology 2010, 109:1140-1147.
4. Scoon GSM, Hopkins WG, Mayhew S, Cotter JD: Effect of post-exercise sauna bathing on the endurance performance of competitive male runners. Journal of Science and Medicine in Sport 2007, 10:259-262.
5. Periard JD, Racinais S, Sawka MN: Adaptations and mechanisms of human heat acclimation: Applications for competitive athletes and sports. Scand J Med Sci Sports 2015, 25 Suppl 1:20-38.
6. Goto M, Okazaki K, Kamijo Y, Ikegawa S, Masuki S, Miyagawa K, Nose H: Protein and carbohydrate supplementation during 5-day aerobic training enhanced plasma volume expansion and thermoregulatory adaptation in young men. Journal of Applied Physiology, 109:1247-1255.

Trent Stellingwerff PhD – The Science of Heat and Hydration

1. Casa DJ, Clarkson PM, Roberts WO: American College of Sports Medicine roundtable on hydration and physical activity: consensus statements. Curr Sports Med Rep 2005, 4:115-127.
2. Wendt D, van Loon LJ, Lichtenbelt WD: Thermoregulation during exercise in the heat: strategies for maintaining health and performance. Sports Med 2007, 37:669-682.
3. Ely MR, Cheuvront SN, Roberts WO, Montain SJ: Impact of weather on marathon-running performance. Medicine and science in sports and exercise 2007, 39:487-493.

ACKNOWLEDGMENTS

I've been fortunate that my professional life has always involved coaching runners. I've never encountered a runner who would not benefit from at least a little bit of coaching. In many cases, the athlete has the ability to be a good runner, and has the determination to be a good runner, but they don't know what to do. In the same way that I work hard to guide runners and help them realize their potential, Zachary Hancock has guided me through the process of editing the raw SMT manuscript into a useful training book for anyone who wants to run a better marathon. After countless revisions, this book is fit for printing. Thanks Zach!

I'm so lucky to have worked with Genevieve Peters on this book. She is smart and thoughtful, and did countless things to make this book a reality. Thank you Genevieve.

When I was writing the outline for the book I was extremely excited about the idea of the Geek Out sections. The contributors to the Geek Out sections are diverse, yet they all are passionate about the sport of running and care a great deal about making this book an important addition to the world of marathon training books. The time and mental energy each spent in writing thoughtfully from their expertise and experience makes this book unlike any other marathon training book that I know of.

Thank you to the readers who took time out of their busy lives to read the manuscript. You helped make this book what it is, and I'm indebted to each of you. And thank you Adam Batliner for a book design that captures the simplicity of the SMT system.

I would be remiss if I didn't thank all of the coaches I've had, going all the way back to my elementary school years. I was blessed with many smart and passionate coaches in a wide range of sports: soccer, tennis, basketball, and summer league track. In college I was fortunate to have Mark Wetmore guide my training, while also opening my mind intellectually in a way that no one else has. It is my aspiration to be as competent, passionate, and caring as all these special coaches have been for me.

Finally, I'd like to acknowledge all of the athletes I've coached up to this point in my life. I work hard to become a better coach each year, and I have indeed improved a great deal over the years, which necessarily implies that the first group of runners I coached at Pratt Community College in Pratt, Kansas suffered through my ignorance as I fumbled through my first years of coaching. To all the Bucky Beavers at Pratt, I wish I could go back in time and coach each of you with the knowledge and the skill that I possess today. And to all of my athletes, both long ago and present, thank you for your energy and dedication and enthusiasm in training, which are inestimable gifts for the serious coach.

ABOUT THE AUTHOR

Jay Johnson has coached collegiate runners, professional runners, and adult runners for more than fifteen years. Jay ran 14:20 for 5,000m and 30:15 for 10,000m as a student-athlete at the University of Colorado, running under the guidance of Mark Wetmore. Jay earned a Master of Science in Kinesiology and Applied Physiology from the University of Colorado, a degree he started working on while running on the varsity cross country team chronicled in the book *Running with the Buffaloes*. Jay has coached three US champions (cross country, indoor track, and road racing), and has helped dozens of adult runners run PRs over distances from 1 mile to 100 hundred miles. Jay is also the director of the Boulder Running Camps, a camp for high school athletes, held each summer on the University of Colorado campus. Jay lives in Arvada, Colorado, with his two daughters, Avery and Louisa. This is his first book.

HOW CAN I SERVE YOU?

You should think of this book as a dialogue between the two of us. I've done my best to communicate to you how you should prepare for your best marathon. This book is a work in progress and I want to hear from you. What questions do you have? Where do you think I can improve the book? How can I serve you? Email me at jay@simplemarathontraining.com. I look forward to hearing from you.

If you enjoyed this book and have two to three minutes, I would sincerely appreciate it if you posted a review on Amazon. My goal is to help as many runners as possible have a great experience with the marathon. The more readers who review *Simple Marathon Training* on Amazon, the more it will be known as a go-to resource for serious runners looking for a smart training book.

I've recorded a guided audio for the fartlek workout in Week One. Go to *SimpleMarathonTraining.com* to download this free audio file. Learning to run by feel is important and this is a great resource to help you do so in your first workout. Finally, go to *SimpleMarathonTraining.com* to download a free PDF with all of the SAM exercises. It is a great tool to help you learn the exercises and routines, though soon you'll have them memorized.

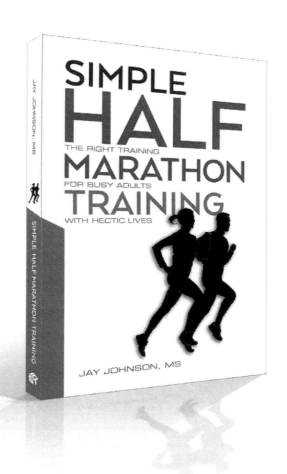

COMING SPRING 2017

SIMPLE HALF MARATHON TRAINING

Visit *SimpleRunningTraining.com* to get the latest
information on these books.

Made in the USA
San Bernardino, CA
20 November 2016